AF823461

Ophthalmic Research

Journal for Research in Experimental and Clinical Ophthalmology

Founded 1970 by O. Hockwin, Bonn, G. Naumann, Hamburg and D.F. Cole, London

Managing Editor

Gijs F.J.M. Vrensen, Amsterdam

Honorary Editor

O. Hockwin, Bonn

Editorial Board

D. Balasubramanian, Hyderabad
A. Bialasiewicz, Hamburg
D. Borchman, Louisville, Ky.
M. Boulton, Manchester
J. Bours, Bonn
B. Ehinger, Lund
D. Fredj-Reygrobellet, Nice
R. van der Gaag, Amsterdam
F.J. Giblin, Rochester, Mich.
J. Graw, Oberschleißheim
K. Green, Augusta, Ga.
B.W. Griffin, Fort Worth, Tex.
S.K. Gupta, New Delhi
N. van Haeringen, Amsterdam
Chr. Hartmann, Berlin
K. Kawasaki, Kanazawa
J.F. Koretz, Troy, N.Y.
Y. de Kozak, Paris
N.H. Lubsen, Nijmegen
C.F. Marfurt, Gary, Ind.
B.R. Masters, Bethesda, Md.
H. Mayer, München
T. Möller-Pedersen, Aarhus
H. Nishigori, Kanagawa
N.N. Osborne, Oxford
C.I. Phillips, Edinburgh
A. Prescott, Dundee
G.L. Ruskell, London
M.F. Saettone, Pisa
K. Sasaki, Ishikawa-Ken
J. Trevithick, London, Ont.
S. Tsukahara, Yamanashi
S. Uga, Kanagawa
A. Wegener, Bonn
J. Weisse, Ingelheim
P. Wiedemann, Leipzig

KARGER

Printed in Switzerland
on acid-free paper by
Thür AG Offsetdruck, Pratteln

Appears bimonthly:
1 volume per year (6 issues)

Ophthalmic Research

Submission: Only original papers written in English are considered and should be sent to:

Dr. Gijs F.J.M. VRENSEN
Department of Morphology
The Netherlands Ophthalmic
Research Institute (NORI)
Meibergdreef 9
1105 AZ Amsterdam
(The Netherlands)
Telephone (020) 566 44 28
Telefax (020) 691 65 21

Manuscripts should be submitted in triplicate (with three sets of illustrations of which one is an original), typewritten double-spaced on one side of the paper, with a wide margin.

Aims and Scope: 'Ophthalmic Research' is meant as an international forum for the dissemination of peer-reviewed information on all aspects of basic research in the field of ophthalmology and visual sciences without refraining from publishing clinical research papers. It specifically aims to elucidate the healthy and pathological functioning of the eye and visual system using the full range of biological, physical and epidemiological research methods.

Types of Papers: (1) The main body of papers to be published will be *'Original Papers'* on experimental research. (2) *'Review Papers'* of up to 30 manuscript pages will be published from invited authors and by direct submission. In both cases the manuscripts will be subject to peer reviewing. Review papers will be published free of charge. (3) *'Short Communications'* of up to 3–4 pages dealing with new original concepts or technical approaches will be published on short notice. (4) *'Ophthalmic Research'* has a tradition in publishing *'Supplements'* which can be published under the responsibility of guest editors. Requests for such supplements should be addressed to the managing editor.

Conditions: All manuscripts are subjected to editorial review. Manuscripts are received with the explicit understanding that they are not under simultaneous consideration by any other publication except an abstract. Submission of an article for publication implies the transfer of the copyright from the author to the publisher upon acceptance. Accepted papers become the permanent property of 'Ophthalmic Research' and may not be reproduced by any means, in whole or in part, without the written consent of the publisher. It is the author's responsibility to obtain permission to reproduce illustrations, tables, etc. from other publications.

Arrangement

Title page: The first page of each paper should indicate the title (main title underlined), the authors' names, and the institute where the work was conducted. A short title for use as running head as well as the full address of the author to whom correspondence should be sent are also required.

Full address: The exact postal address complete with postal code must be given at the bottom of the title page. Please also supply Phone, Fax, and E-mail numbers.

Key words: For indexing purposes, a list of 3 – 10 key words in English is essential.

Abstract: Each paper needs an abstract of up to 10 lines.

Small type: Paragraphs which can or must be set in smaller type (case histories, test methods, etc.) should be indicated with a 'p' (petit) in the margin on the left-hand side.

Footnotes: Avoid footnotes. When essential, they are numbered consecutively and typed at the foot of the appropriate page.

Tables and illustrations: Tables and illustrations (both numbered in Arabic numerals) should be prepared on separate sheets. Tables require a heading and figures a legend, also prepared on a separate sheet. For the reproduction of illustrations, only good drawings and original photographs can be accepted; negatives or photocopies cannot be used. Due to technical reasons, figures with a screen background should not be submitted. When possible, group several illustrations on one block for reproduction (max. size 144 × 196 mm) or provide crop marks. On the back of each illustration, indicate its number, the author's name, and 'top' with a soft pencil. Photographs of microscopic preparations should be labeled with the magnification scale, e.g. 1 μm.

Color illustrations: Up to 6 color illustrations per page can now be integrated with the text at the reduced price of CHF 600.– / USD 545.00 per page. Color illustrations are reproduced at the author's expense.

References: In the text identify references by Arabic numerals [in square brackets]. Material submitted for publication but not yet accepted should be noted as 'unpublished data' and not be included in the reference list. The list of references should include only those publications which are cited in the text. Do not alphabetize; number references in the order in which they are first mentioned in the text. The surnames of the authors followed by initials should be given. There should be no punctuation other than a comma to separate the authors. Cite all authors, 'et al' is not sufficient. Abbreviate journal names according to the Index Medicus system. (Also see International Committee of Medical Journal Editors: Uniform requirements for manuscripts submitted to biomedical journals. Br Med J 1988;296:401–405.)

Examples

(a) Papers published in periodicals: Kauffman HF, van der Heide S, Beaumont F, Blok H, de Vries K: Class-specific antibody determination against *Aspergillus fumigatus* by means of the enzyme-linked immunosorbent assay. III. Comparative study: IgG, IgA, IgM ELISA titers, precipitating antibodies and IgE binding after fractionation of the antigen. Int Arch Allergy Appl Immunol 1986;80:300–306.

(b) Monographs: Matthews DE, Farewell VT: Using and Understanding Medical Statistics. Basel, Karger, 1985.

(c) Edited books: Hardy WD Jr, Essex M: FeLV-induced feline acquired immune deficiency syndrome: A model for human AIDS; in Klein E (ed): Acquired Immunodeficiency Syndrome. Prog Allergy. Basel, Karger, 1986, vol 37, pp 353–376.

Further details: Authors may consult our leaflet 'Rules for the Preparation of Manuscripts', available on request from the Publisher, S. Karger AG, P.O. Box, CH – 4009 Basel (Switzerland).

Page charges: There is no page charge for papers of 3 or fewer printed pages (including tables, illustrations and references). Each additional complete or partial page is charged to the author at CHF 380.– / USD 300.00 / DEM 460.–. The allotted size of a paper is equal to approx. 8 manuscript pages (including tables, illustrations and references). Authors of manuscripts that will exceed this allotted size are requested to submit, together with the manuscript, a written statement of their willingness to accept page charges.

Galley proofs: Unless indicated otherwise, galley proofs are sent to the first-named author and should be returned with the least possible delay. Alterations made in galley proofs, other than the correction of printer's errors, are charged to the author. No page proofs are supplied.

Reprints: Order forms and a price list are sent with the galley proofs. Orders submitted after the issue is printed are subject to considerably higher prices. Allow five weeks from date of publication for delivery of reprints.

KARGER
E-Mail karger@karger.ch
Fax + 41 61 306 12 34
http://www.karger.ch

General Information
http://www.karger.ch/journals/ore/oredes.htm

Ophthalmic Research

Publication data: 'Ophthalmic Research' is published 6 times annually. Volume 28 with 6 issues appears in 1996.
Subscription rates: Subscriptions run for a full calendar year. Prices are given per volume.
Personal subscription:

Subscription	+ *postage and handling*
CHF 357.60	+ CHF 22.10 Europe
CHF 357.60	+ CHF 33.60 Overseas
USD 274.80	+ USD 22.10

(Must be in the name of, billed to, and paid by an individual. Order must be marked 'personal subscription'.)
Institutional subscription:

Subscription	+ *postage and handling*
CHF 596.–	+ CHF 27.60 Europe
CHF 596.–	+ CHF 42.– Overseas
USD 458.00	+ USD 27.60

Airmail postage: CHF 36.–, USD 30.00. (Extra per volume.)
Discount subscription prices:
Association for Eye Research;
Association for Research and Vision in Ophthalmology.
Advertising: Correspondence and rate requests should be addressed to the Publisher.
Change of address: Both old and new address should be sent to the subscription source.

Microforms: Please direct all enquiries and orders to:
University Microfilms Inc.
300 North Zeeb Road, P.O. Box 1346
Ann Arbor, MI 48106-1346 (USA)
Subscription orders: Orders can be placed at agencies, bookstores, directly with the Publisher S. Karger AG, P.O. Box, CH – 4009 Basel (Switzerland)
or with any of the following distributors:
Deutschland: S. Karger GmbH, Postfach
D – 79095 Freiburg
France: Librairie Luginbühl
36, bd de Latour-Maubourg
F–75007 Paris
Great Britain, Ireland: S. Karger Publishers
11 Ravenscroft Road
Beckenham, Kent BR3 4TP
USA: S. Karger Publishers, Inc.
26 West Avon Road, P.O. Box 529
Farmington, CT 06085
India, Bangladesh, Sri Lanka:
S. Karger India Subscription Agency
B – 5/132 Safdarjung Enclave
New Delhi-110029
Japan: Katakura Libri, Inc.
Take 1 Bldg, 2nd Floor
4-5-7 Yushima, Bunkyo-ku
Tokyo 113

Single issues and back volumes: Information can be obtained through the Publisher.
Bibliographic indices: This journal is regularly listed in bibliographic services, including *Current Contents®*.
Copying: This journal has been registered with the Copyright Clearance Center (CCC), as indicated by the code appearing on the first page of each article. For readers in the US, this code signals consent for copying of articles for personal or internal use, or for the personal or internal use of specific clients, provided that the stated fee is paid per copy directly to Copyright Clearance Center, Inc., 222 Rosewood Drive, Danvers, MA 01923 (USA). A copy of the first page of the article must accompany payment. Consent does not extend to copying for general distribution, for promotion, for creating new works, or for resale. In these cases, specific written permission must be obtained from the copyright owner, S. Karger AG, P.O. Box, CH–4009 Basel (Switzerland).
KARGER
E-Mail karger@karger.ch
Fax + 41 61 306 12 34
http://www.karger.ch

Successfully answers the needs of congress organizers

Gideon Rivlin

Guide to Organizing an International Scientific Conference

Whether you are organizing a scientific conference for under 400 participants or attempting to attract upwards of 5,000 delegates, this step-by-step guide will be your essential desk-top companion.

Contents
- The First Ten Steps
- Administration, Secretariat and Manpower
- Promotion and Sponsorship
- Halls and Technical Arrangements
- Registration
- Printing
- Budget
- The Commercial Exhibition
- Social Events
- Services at the Conference Site
- Tourism
- Dealing with What Can Go Wrong
- Evaluating Your Conference: The Conference Effectiveness Study
- Future Conference Technology
- Afterword

Fields of Interest: General Medicine, Communication, Documentation

Rivlin, G. (Tel Aviv)
Guide to Organizing an International Scientific Conference
X + 94 p., 11 fig., 1 tab., soft cover, 1995
CHF 78.– / DEM 93.– / USD 68.00
Prices subject to change
DEM price for Germany, USD price for USA only
ISBN 3–8055–6151–2
Ask about our special prices for orders of ten or more copies!

KARGER

KI 96425

Everything you've always wanted to know about statistics in one highly-recommended book

David E. Matthews
Vernon T. Farewell

Using and Understanding Medical Statistics

3rd, revised edition

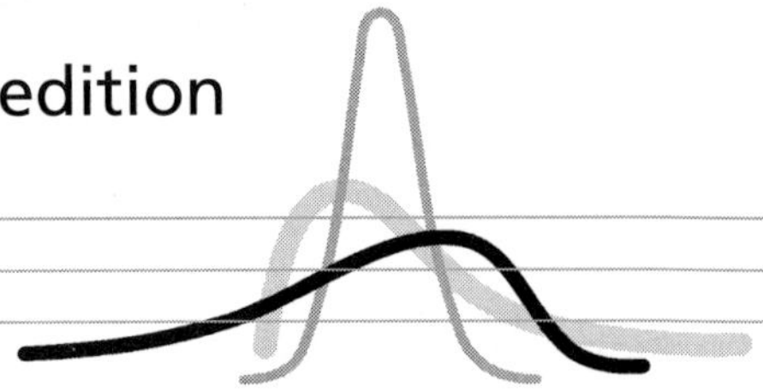

Contents

- Basic Concepts
- Tests of Significance
- Fisher's Test for 2×2 Contingency Tables
- Approximate Significance Tests for Contingency Tables
- Some Warnings Concerning 2×2 Tables
- Kaplan-Meier or 'Actuarial' Survival Curves
- The Log-Rank or Mantel-Haenszel Test for the Comparison of Survival Curves
- An Introduction to the Normal Distribution
- Analyzing Normally Distributed Data
- Linear Regression Models for Medical Data
- Binary Logistic Regression
- Proportional Hazards Regression
- The Analysis of Longitudinal Data
- Data Analysis
- The Question of Sample Size
- The Design of Clinical Trials
- Further Comments Regarding Clinical Trials
- Epidemiological Applications

Since the last edition of this book was published, major developments in computer technology have affected both the practice of medicine and the methods of analyzing medical data. These advances make the focus of this revised edition – understanding many of the statistical methods that are used in modern medical studies – all the more important. Two new chapters have been added by the authors. One provides readers with an introduction to the analysis of longitudinal data. The other augments previous material concerning the design of clinical trials, exploring topics such as the use of surrogate markers, multiple outcomes, equivalence trials, and the planning of efficacy-toxicity studies. In addition to providing new information and fine-tuning the rest of the book, the authors have reorganized the final six chapters so that the topics build, naturally, on each other. This latest edition is highly recommended both as an excellent introduction to medical statistics and as a valuable tool in explaining the more complex statistical methods and techniques used today.

Matthews, D.E. (Waterloo, Ont.); Farewell, V.T. (London)
Using and Understanding Medical Statistics
3rd, revised edition
XIV + 246 p., 31 fig., 86 tab., hard cover, 1996
CHF 40.– / DEM 48.– / USD 35.00
Prices subject to change
DEM price for Germany, USD price for USA only
ISBN 3–8055–6276–4

Fields of Interest: General Medicine, Social Medicine; Communication, Medical Statistics, Epidemiology

KI 96445

KARGER

International Forum on Advanced Techniques in Lens and Cataract Research

7th Scheimpflug Club
Meeting
Kanazawa, June 6–8, 1995

Editors
K. Sasaki, Uchinada, Japan
O. Hockwin, Bonn, Germany

81 figures, 2 in color, 10 tables, 1996

KARGER

S. Karger
Medical and Scientific Publishers
Basel · Freiburg · Paris · London
New York · New Delhi · Bangkok
Singapore · Tokyo · Sydney

Drug Dosage
The authors and the publisher have exerted every effort to ensure that drug selection and dosage set forth in this text are in accord with current recommendations and practice at the time of publication. However, in view of ongoing research, changes in government regulations, and the constant flow of information relating to drug therapy and drug reactions, the reader is urged to check the package insert for each drug for any change in indications and dosage and for added warnings and precautions. This is particularly important when the recommended agent is a new and/or infrequently employed drug.

All rights reserved.
No part of this publication may be translated into other languages, reproduced or utilized in any form or by any means, electronic or mechanical, including photocopying, recording, microcopying, or by any information storage and retrieval system, without permission in writing from the publisher or, in the case of photocopying, direct payment of a specified fee to the Copyright Clearance Center (see 'Information for Readers and Subscribers').

© Copyright 1996 by S. Karger AG,
P.O. Box, CH–4009 Basel (Switzerland)
Printed in Switzerland on acid-free paper by
Thür AG Offsetdruck, Pratteln
ISBN 3–8055–6379–5

Ophthalmic Research

Vol. 28, Supplement 2, 1996

Contents

KARGER

E-Mail karger@karger.ch
Fax + 41 61 306 12 34
http://www.karger.ch

© 1996 S. Karger AG, Basel

The list of contents is available at:
http://www.karger.ch/journals/ore/orecont.htm

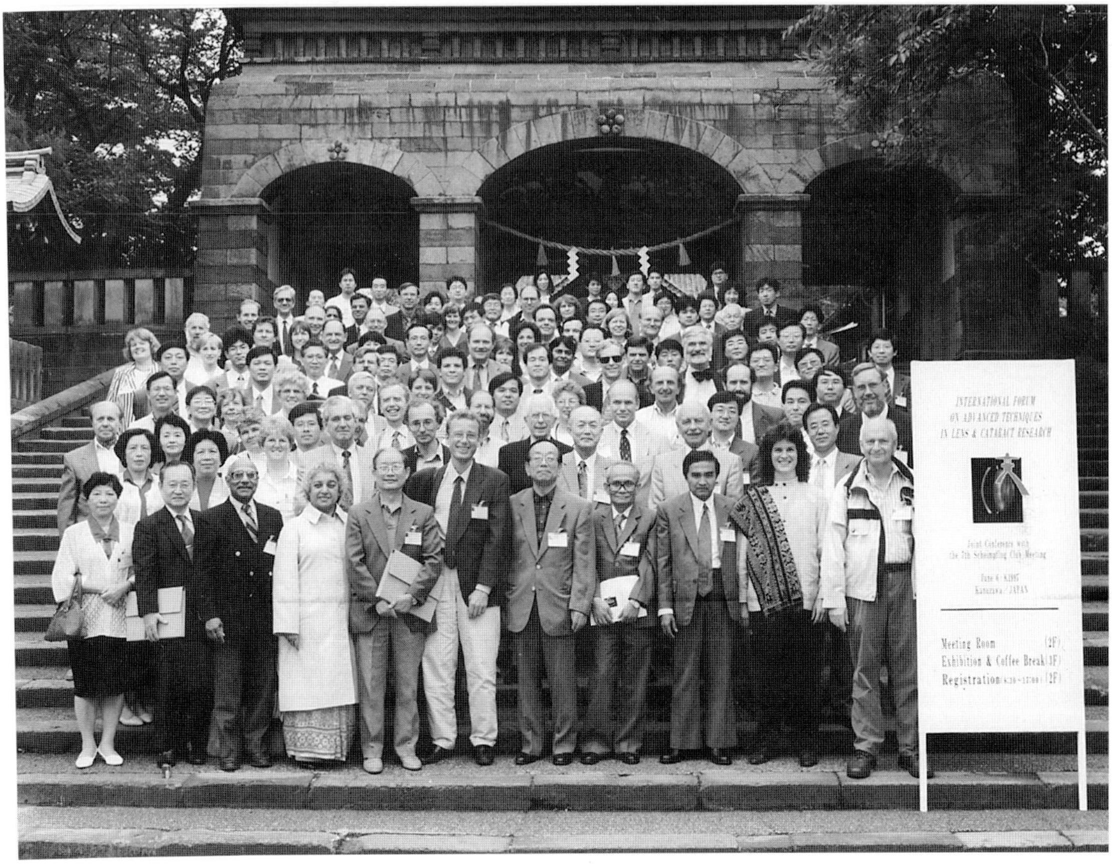
INTERNATIONAL FORUM
ON ADVANCED TECHNIQUES
IN LENS & CATARACT RESEARCH
Meeting Room (2F)
Exhibition & Coffee Break (3F)
Registration (2F)

Foreword

Kazuyuki Sasaki, MD

Department of Ophthalmology,
Kanazawa Medical University,
Uchinada, Japan

The Scheimpflug Club Meeting was initiated by Prof. Otto Hockwin (Bonn, Germany), Prof. Sidney Lerman (Atlanta, USA) and myself in 1985. Since that time, a meeting has been held nearly every 2 years. During the 1980s Scheimpflug-related studies were only discussed by limited research groups, in particular those concerning the lens. However, recent camera systems applying computer-assisted techniques have widened the field of its application. Consequently, topics discussed in recent Scheimpflug Club Meetings have become varied. The 7th meeting, which was held in Kanazawa, Japan, from June 6th to 8th, was entitled International Forum on Advanced Techniques in Lens and Cataract Research, with a total of 105 papers presented. Of the above papers, except UV-related cataract epidemiological studies, 21 are published in supplement 2 of Ophthalmic Research, volume 28, 1996. I believe the readers may acquire useful information from this supplement for their research.

As editors of this supplement, we are grateful to the chief editor of Ophthalmic Research and S. Karger AG for giving us the opportunity to publish this supplement.

Ophthalmic Research

Ophthalmic Res 1996;28(suppl 2):1–4

Physiological Influence on Ocular Photometry

A Review

Therese DeMel[a]
Peter W.J. Dekker[b]
Anton Lechner[b]
Yves C.A. Robert[b]
Phillip Hendrickson[a]

University Eye Clinics of
[a] Basel and
[b] Zurich, Switzerland

Key Words
Ocular photometry
Contrast transfer
Lens
Opacification

Abstract
During the development of the ocular photometer (OPM) since 1983, we have considered several physical and physiological factors that could potentially influence the measurement and its results. Attention has been given to respiratory, circulatory, and intraocular pressure provocations, and numerous publications document the influences or lack thereof. Most recently, the authors conducted a simple reproducibility study with only 1 observer and 1 subject. Measurement of the same 2 retinal sites during a 3-week period yielded no statistically significant differences, even under relatively extreme temperature conditions. Thus, changes in readings with the OPM may be considered due to variations within the eye, such as cataract. Thus, increase in lens density may be directly and correctly expressed by dual-site measurement of retinal brightness, resulting in the contrast transfer ratio.

Introduction and History

In 1983, using a modified Zeiss fundus camera with a light-sensitive diode in the image plane, Robert made the first direct measurement of fundus brightness and, thus, introduced the method of ocular photometry [1, 2]. The first application of the device, the ocular photometer (OPM) was in the analysis of the distribution of brightness around the vital rim of the papilla. Interestingly, the temporal rims of right papillas were consistently the brightest of the 4 sites measured (temporal OD, nasal OD, nasal OS, temporal OS) [3].

KARGER

E-Mail karger@karger.ch
Fax + 41 61 306 12 34
http://www.karger.ch

© 1996 S. Karger AG, Basel
0030–3747/96/0288–0001$10.00/0

Therese DeMel, OPS
Photography Department
University Eye Clinic
PO Box
CH–4012 Basel (Switzerland)

Respiratory and Circulatory Provocation

That same year (1983) we investigated the possible influence of physiological parameters on the measurements [4]. In 6 German shepherd dogs, vital parameters of respiration and circulation were strongly manipulated while the OPM documented papillary brightness and vessel diameters. Under extreme manipulation of both parameters, the brightness and the vessel diameters remained unchanged.

Contrast Transfer through the Ocular Media

In 1985 we sought to quantify opacification of the ocular media. Opacification reduces the optical performance of the ocular media with regard to their ability to transfer contrast from object space into image space, that is onto the retina. This phenomenon is easily understood [5]: A square-wave contrast pattern (black and white bars) consists of a fundamental sine wave of the same spatial frequency, F, augmented by sine waves of increasing frequency (3F, 5F, 7F...nF) but decreasing energy. The fundamental waves gradually develop corners until they become squared off. Indeed, these finest, high-frequency sine waves give a square-wave pattern its sharp 90° edges.

When a square-wave pattern is imaged through an imperfect optical system, such as a cataractous eye, those sine waves with the weakest energy and highest frequency are the first to be lost. As a result, both the amplitudes of brightness and darkness as well as the sharpness of the contrast edges are reduced, and, in cataract, such reduction in bright and dark portions of the Snellen E results in a lower visual acuity (VA).

By reversing the direction of contrast transfer (traditional ophthalmoscopic view) and measuring a *bright* site, the papilla, and a *dark* site, the macula, through the same optical system (here the eye), we can quantify its optical efficiency, which in turn is directly correlated with the VA.

Such sequential brightness measurement of 2 retinal sites is provided by a second-generation OPM prototype codeveloped with Haag-Streit (Bern, Switzerland), and the 2 values were incorporated into a ratio of relative brightness, the constrast transfer ratio (CTR). In two separate trials in Basel and Zurich [6], we measured the CTR in 80 persons of varying VA with no ocular pathology, finding a direct correlation between the CTR value and the VA ($r^2 = 0.52$, $r = 0.72$, $p < 0.001$).

Comparison of preoperative and postoperative CTR and VAs in 40 implant surgery patients showed parallel improvement in the respective parameters (CTR from 1.39 ± 0.42 to 1.95 ± 0.53; VA from 0.11 ± 0.05 to 0.70 ± 0.11; $p < 0.001$).

Papillary Brightness under Intraocular Pressure Provocation

Since the introduction of the second-generation prototype in 1985, manipulation of various local and systemic parameters was conducted to analyze their potential influence on brightness results. First of these was a locally induced abrupt increase in intraocular pressure (IOP) [7]. The provocation was implemented by means of a suction cup placed on the conjunctiva. Differences in papillary brightness were striking. This is due to evacuation of red blood cells from the capillaries of the papilla. Normally, blue and green wavelengths are absorbed by the red blood cells. After a certain time of provocation, perfusion breaks down, the red blood cells are pressed out, and the blue and green light is reflected, adding to the total brightness. Clinically, the papilla is seen to become pale.

Latency times (that is, the delay between onset of IOP elevation and breakdown of papillary perfusion) were obviously greater in normals (2.39 ± 0.68) than in glaucoma patients (0.64 ± 0.25) [8, 9]. This effect was consistently different in the two groups. Such differences in latency times provide a new circulatory parameter, which we term dynamic provoked circulatory response.

In the University Eye Clinic Zurich, Professor Robert's team continues to pursue investigation of the relationship between OPM measurements and certain other physical and physiological parameters. The results are the focus of an article submitted for publication elsewhere.

Reproducibility

In a reproducibility study, the same fundus sites in the right eye of one author (P.H.) were measured daily at the same time of day by the same examiner (T.D.), using a fundus sketch for orientation. The results were reassuring: Under constant room temperature conditions (+19 °C), the CTR values remain stable (1.88 ± 0.03). Even when the subject was exposed to outside cold (+2 °C) for 30 min before measurement, only a nonsignificant ($p = 0.12$) tendency towards higher values was noted.

Conclusion

In summary, investigations with the OPM have shown that, even under relatively extreme physical and physiological conditions (except abrupt IOP elevation), measurement of the brightness of individual fundus sites remains essentially uninfluenced and highly reproducible. Such reproducibility encourages us to pursue further applications of the OPM (beyond the scope of this present article): in distinguishing between elective and indicated cataract surgery [6, 10–12]; in establishing the contribution of lens quality to poor visual-field results [13]; in directly evaluating the effect on perfusion of anesthetics [7–9] and in providing the internist a means of objectively and noninvasively determining perfusion alterations in response to various medications [14–16].

References

1 Hendrickson Ph, Robert Y: Direkte Messung der Papillenhelligkeit. Klin Monatsbl Augenheilkd 1984;184: 357–358.

2 Hendrickson Ph, Robert Y, Stöckli HP: Principles of photometry of the papilla. Arch Ophthalmol 1984;102: 1704–1707.

3 Robert Y, Hendrickson Ph: Color appearance of the papilla in normal and glaucomatous eyes: A photopapillometric study. Arch Ophthalmol 1984;102:1772–1775.

4 Robert Y, Hendrickson Ph, Bläss J, Gerber H: Respiratory and circulatory influence on photopapillometry. Graefes Arch Clin Exp Ophthalmol 1986;224:96–100.

5 Hendrickson Ph, Robert Y: Klinische Bestimmung des funktionellen Trübungsgrades einer Katarakt: Theorie und Technik. Klin Monatsbl Augenheilkd 1986;188:421–424.

6 Hendrickson Ph, Robert Y: Contrast transfer ratio in normal, cataractous, and intraocular implant lenses: A clinical photopapillometric study. Graefes Arch Clin Exp Ophthalmol 1986;224:191–194.

7 Robert Y, Hendrickson Ph: Photometry of the optic disc; in Lambrou GN, Greve EL (eds): Ocular Blood Flow. Amstelveen, Kugler & Ghedini, 1989, pp 167–172.

8 Robert Y, Hendrickson Ph: Dynamic provoked circulatory response (DPCR) of the papilla. New Trends Ophthalmol 1986;1:253–257.
9 Robert Y, Steiner D, Hendrickson Ph: Papillary circulation dynamics in glaucoma. Graefes Arch Clin Exp Ophthalmol 1989;227:436–439.
10 Robert Y, Hendrickson Ph: Die Quantifizierung der Katarakt an der Spaltlampe. Klin Monatsbl Augenheilkd 1988;192:406–408.
11 Hendrickson Ph, Robert Y: La mesure de l'opacité des milieux de l'œil avec l'OPM (Ocular Photometer de Haag-Streit). Ophtalmologie (Paris) 1991;5:19–21.
12 Hoppeler Th, Hendrickson Ph, Robert Y: Subjektive Funktion und 'Pap/Mak'-Verhältnis bei geringgradiger Medientrübung. Klin Monatsbl Augenheilkd 1988;192:400–402.
13 Robert Y, Hendrickson Ph: The influence of beta-blocking agents with and without intrinsic sympathomimetic activity on the capillary blood volume of the optic nerve head. Doc Ophthalmol Proc Ser 1985;43:103–109.
14 Hendrickson Ph, Robert Y: Beurteilung der Wirksamkeit von β-Blokkern am Auge. Klin Monatsbl Augenheilkd 1985;186:498–499.
15 Robert Y, Grauwiler Th, Hendrickson Ph, Brunner HR: Die Autoregulation der Papillengefässe und ihr Verhalten unter Halothan. Klin Monatsbl Augenheilkd 1988;192:117–121.
16 Yüksel Y, Thölen H, Meier R, Hendrickson Ph, Robert Y: Über die Autoregulation der Aderhaut. Klin Monatsbl Augenheilkd 1992;200:343–345.

Ophthalmic Research

Ophthalmic Res 1996;28(suppl 2):5–10

Nuclear Magnetic Resonance Studies of Sugar Metabolism in the Human Infant Lens

Hong-Ming Cheng[a]
Jing Xiong[a]
Shinjiro Hirose[a]
Hiromasa Igarashi[a]
Tatsuo Hirose[b]

[a] NMR Research, Howe Laboratory of Ophthalmology, Harvard Medical School, and Massachusetts Eye and Ear Infirmary, and
[b] Retina Associates, Boston, Mass., USA

Key Words
Human infant lens
Retinopathy of prematurity
Nuclear magnetic resonance spectroscopy
Sugar metabolism
Hexose monophosphate shunt
Polyol pathway

Abstract
We investigated sugar metabolism in lenses isolated from infants with stage-5 retinopathy of prematurity (ROP). The lenses were incubated in ^{13}C-labeled glucose (35.5 m*M*) or galactose (30 m*M*) for 24 h at 37.5 °C. Six to 8 lenses were pooled for each experiment. ^{13}C-nuclear magnetic resonance spectroscopy was then performed on perchloric acid extracts of these lenses. Active aldose metabolism was indicated by the production of lactate. However, neither sorbitol nor dulcitol was detected. On the other hand, an experimental aldose reductase inhibitor, sorbinil, caused a decrease in the hexose monophosphate shunt activity suggesting an active polyol pathway. Both polyols therefore appeared to have been metabolized further. In addition, galactose metabolism was unique in that it not only involved a galactose → glucose epimerization, but also a direct galactose → ribose conversion, and a production of galactose-3-phosphate. Although it is possible that the ROP lenses have adapted to oxidative stress during the postnatal high-oxygen incubation for premature infants, we believe the observed sugar metabolism is representative of the developing human lens.

KARGER

E-Mail karger@karger.ch
Fax + 41 61 306 12 34
http://www.karger.ch

© 1996 S. Karger AG, Basel

Dr. Hong-Ming Cheng
Howe Laboratory of Ophthalmology
243 Charles Street
Boston, MA 02114 (USA)

Introduction

Current understanding of lens metabolism is based to a large extent on animal models. The lack of intact normal human lenses has restricted comparative studies. The lens supply situation has worsened since the introduction of phacoemulsification/extracapsular-cataract surgery. We now have a unique opportunity to study infant lenses removed intracapsularly during open-sky vitrectomy for the treatment of stage-5 retinopathy of prematurity (ROP). These cryoextracted lenses, although not as trauma-free as freshly excised animal lenses, do show active metabolism. We examined aldose metabolism through glycolysis, hexose monophosphate shunt (HMPS), and the polyol pathway using ^{13}C-nuclear magnetic resonance (^{13}C-NMR) spectroscopy previously developed for the lens [1]. To increase NMR detection sensitivity, we pooled 6–8 lenses for each experiment. The results are different from animal lens studies in several aspects, for example, polyol pathway activation, galactose→glucose/ribose conversion, and a possible galactose-3-phosphate production. These results and the significance of the findings are presented in this report.

Materials and Methods

Human infant lenses (ages < 2 years, the majority <1 year) were extracted intracapsularly with a cryoprobe as part of the open-sky vitrectomy. All adhering tissues were carefully removed. The lenses were clear with intact capsules; some showed slight capsular haze but none exhibited frank cortical, nuclear or subcapsular opacities as those seen in senile cataracts. They were stored at 0–4 °C for up to 4 h, transported from the operating room to the laboratory, and incubated in TC199-bicarbonate medium containing ^{13}C-labeled glucose or galactose (medium osmolarity = 300 mosm with pH = 7.4 maintained by 95% air, 5% CO_2). ^{13}C-labeled glucose (at carbon-2) and galactose (at carbon-1) were purchased from Cambridge Isotope Laboratories, Woburn, Mass., USA. Sorbinil, an experimental aldose reductase (AR) inhibitor, was provided by Pfizer Central Research, Groton, Conn., USA. Each lens (about 0.11 g wet weight) was incubated in 10 ml medium at 37.5 °C in a sealed incubation vial. After 24 h the lens was removed from the medium, blotted dry on Whatman No. 1 filter paper, and immediately frozen with liquid N_2 and stored at –80 °C. Six to 8 lenses were pooled and perchloric acid extraction was performed at liquid N_2 temperature using a mortar and pestle. Details of the extraction procedure were described by González et al. [2] except that the final lyophilizates were reconstituted with H_2O (at 1 g lens wet weight/ml) instead of D_2O. The incubating media were also saved and kept at –80 °C until use. No kinetic studies were done, owing to the difficulty in coordinating surgical schedule and NMR machine time.

^{13}C-NMR spectroscopy was performed with a Bruker MSL400 spectrometer using a 10-mm broadband probe. The spectra were acquired with proton decoupling and the following parameters included: sweep frequency, 100.613 MHz; 32 K data points; sweep width, 20,000 Hz; pulse duration, 11 μs (90°); interpulse delay, 5 s, and 20 Hz line broadening. Identification of resonances was based on literature chemical-shift values and when necessary, confirmed with authentic compounds.

Results

Glucose Metabolism

A 24-hour incubation of the lenses with 35.5 m*M* $^{13}C_2$-glucose showed only $^{13}C_2$-lactate but no sorbitol; however, large resonances of a carbonyl group, $^{13}C{=}O$ (162 ppm), and a $^{13}C{-}H$ group (82 ppm) appeared (fig. 1a). The signal intensities of lactate and these 2 resonances were similar.

We further tested whether the lens responded to an interference with AR activity. The lenses were incubated in 35.5 m*M* $^{13}C_2$-glucose in the presence of 40 μ*M* sorbinil. The ^{13}C metabolite pattern was now entirely different: the 162- and 82-ppm resonances were substantially reduced and $^{13}C_3$-lactate appeared (fig. 1b). This result indicates that the lens glucose metabolism responded to the AR inhibitor.

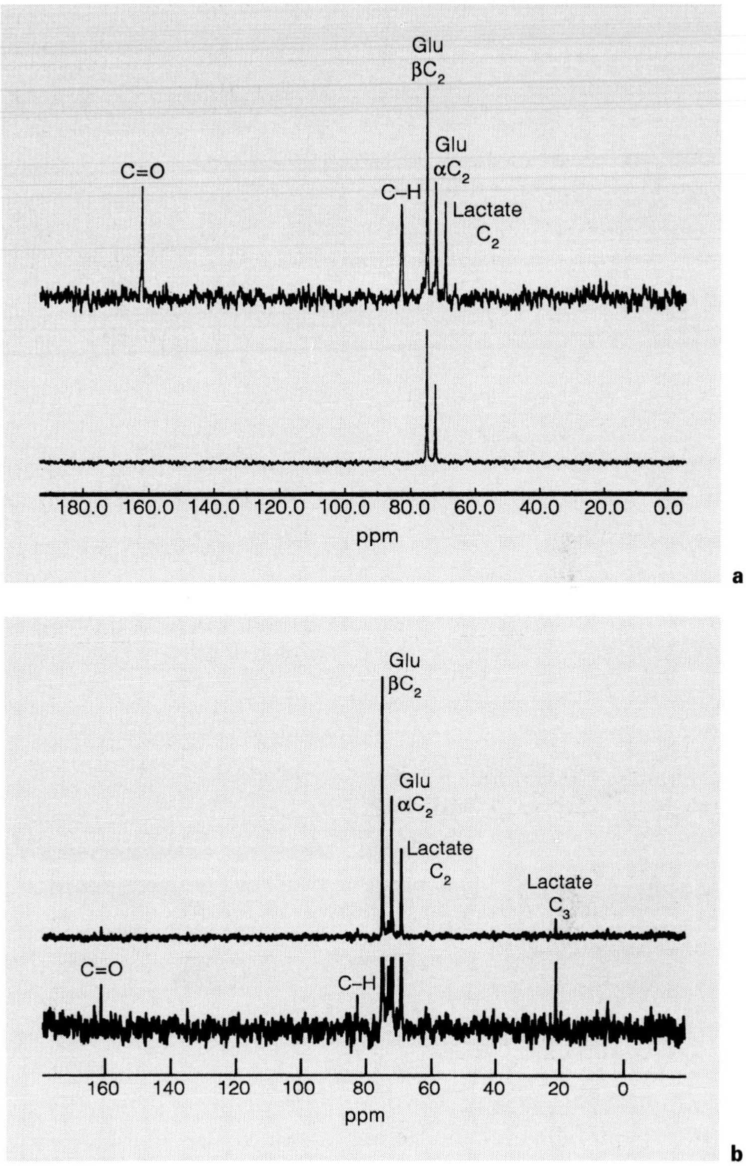

Fig. 1. ^{13}C-NMR spectra of lenses incubated in (**a**) 35.5 m*M* $^{13}C_2$-glucose: (top) lens spectrum; (bottom) incubating medium, and (**b**) 35.5 m*M* $^{13}C_2$-glucose + 40 μ*M* sorbinil (top) lens; (bottom) the expanded version of the lens spectrum. The lenses were incubated at 37 °C for 24 h. Glu = Glucose.

Galactose Metabolism

The lenses were incubated in 30 m*M* $^{13}C_1$-galactose in the presence of 5.5 m*M* unlabeled glucose for 24 h. Based on animal studies, dulcitol is not further metabolized and therefore should accumulate in the lens [3]. However, no dulcitol was detected, although both $^{13}C_1$- and $^{13}C_3$-lactate (178 and 21 ppm, respectively) appeared (fig. 2a). Sorbinil was then added to the medium; surprisingly, the C=O group (162 ppm) now appeared (fig. 2b). This suggests a decrease in the HMPS activity because

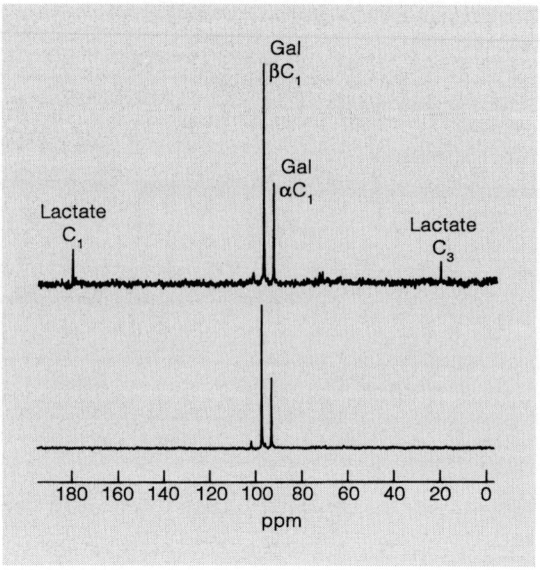

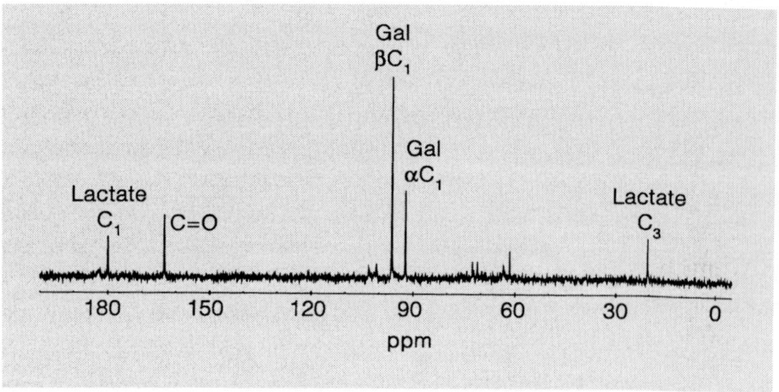

Fig. 2. a 30 m*M* $^{13}C_1$-galactose + 5.5 m*M* unenriched glucose. Top = lens; bottom = medium. **b** 30 m*M* $^{13}C_1$-galactose + 5.5 m*M* unenriched glucose + 40 μ*M* sorbinil. The incubation conditions were identical to those in figure 1. Gal = Galactose.

the unlabeled glucose no longer entered the HMPS, thus allowing the $^{13}C{=}O$ resonance to be seen.

Discussion

There appears to be a high degree of glucose flux through the HMPS. When $^{13}C_2$-glucose is metabolized through the HMPS, the carbon-2 label is redistributed in two steps. Step 1: it first re-emerges at the carbon-1 of pentoses and eventually the carbon-1, -3 and -5 of glucose-6-phosphate (with $^{13}C_5$ derived in part from $^{13}C_2$-glyceraldehyde-3-phosphate generated from the Embden-Meyerhof pathway), and step 2: when $^{13}C_{1,3,5}$-glucose-6-phosphate recycles through the HMPS, C-1 is again lost, the label now appears at carbon-2 and -4 of pentoses.

Evidence of step 2 is shown in figure 1a: prominent resonances of a carbonyl group $^{13}C{=}O$ (162 ppm), and a ^{13}C–H group (82 ppm) appeared. Based on preliminary studies, this C=O group appears to be the C-2 of xylulose and the C–H group that of the C-4 of ribose.

These results are consistent with the metabolism of $^{13}C_2$-glucose through the HMPS mediated through ribose, that is, after decarboxylation, the ^{13}C label now is located at C-1 of ribose (step 1) which then further proceeded through the HMPS (step 2).

Figure 1b shows tht the inclusion of an AR inhibitor with $^{13}C_2$-glucose in the incubating medium lowered the signal intensities of both the ^{13}C–H (82 ppm) and the ^{13}C=O (162 ppm) resonances, but $^{13}C_3$-lactate now appeared. Because of this response, we conclude that the AR/polyol pathway must have been inhibited. The glucose flow through the HMPS on the other hand remains uninterrupted because of the presence of $^{13}C_3$-lactate. Its presence indicates recycling of glucose ($^{13}C_2$-glucose → $^{13}C_1$-glucose-6-phosphate) through the HMPS (step 1). This mode of glucose recycling also has been observed in animal lenses [4].

The results above additionally imply an extremely active AR/polyol pathway. The lack of accumulation of sorbitol therefore is due to a high sorbitol turnover through fructose and/or sorbitol-3-phosphate [5].

Galactose metabolism is unique in the human infant lens. Production of ^{13}C-lactate from ^{13}C-galactose is not seen in the rat lens [3], whereas in the human infant lens, both $^{13}C_1$- and $^{13}C_3$-lactate were produced. The latter indicates a high degree of rearrangement of carbon skeletons. There are three possible mechanisms: (1) galactose → glucose epimerization – this explains the production of $^{13}C_3$-lactate; (2) a direct $^{13}C_1$-galactose → $^{13}C_1$-ribose conversion – this allows the production of ^{13}C=O, and (3) the production of the 3-phosphates of galactose and/or dulcitol – this is the only possibility for the formation of $^{13}C_1$-lactate.

If the epimerization process alone takes place, the $^{13}C_1$ label will be lost through the HMPS decarboxylation. Clearly this is not the case, because in order to form ^{13}C=O, a carryover of the $^{13}C_1$ label of galactose into ribose must take place. We therefore propose a direct galactose → ribose conversion.

Evidence for galactose-3-phosphate production is now lacking, although the 3-phosphorylase mechanism exists in the human lens because of the presence of sorbitol-3-phosphate [6]. Phosphorylation of galactose and/or dulcitol at carbon-3, however, remains the only plausible explanation for the retention of the ^{13}C at carbon-1 of lactate which is derived from glucose-3-phosphate epimerized from galactose-3-phosphate and/or the breakdown of dulcitol-3-phosphate similar to that of sorbitol-3-phosphate [5].

The response of the lens to sorbinil, i.e., with an increase in ^{13}C=O (fig. 2b), is indicative of a lowered glucose flux through the HMPS, because a high glucose flow would have diluted the ^{13}C=O label. This response again implies active polyol pathway activity and that dulcitol is actively being metabolized.

Aldose metabolism in human infant lenses apparently is quite different from that in rat and rabbit lenses and is summarized below:

(1) $^{13}C_2$-glucose → $^{13}C_2$-lactate + $^{13}C_2$-xylulose-5-P + $^{13}C_4$-ribose-5-P (fig. 1a),
$^{13}C_2$-glucose + sorbinil → $^{13}C_2$-lactate + $^{13}C_3$-lactate (fig. 1b), and

(2) $^{13}C_1$-galactose + unlabeled glucose → $^{13}C_1$-lactate + $^{13}C_3$-lactate (fig. 2a),
$^{13}C_1$-galactose + unlabeled glucose + sorbinil → $^{13}C_1$-lactate + $^{13}C_3$-lactate + $^{13}C_2$-xylulose-5-P (fig. 2b).

Although the metabolic pattern described above is derived from lenses of human infants with stage-5 ROP, it is unlikely that this pattern is present only in ROP lenses. The difference between normal and ROP lenses, if any, will be largely a matter of the extent in their responses to oxidative stress. Further, the presence of AR but little sorbitol in the intact human lens and human lens epithelial cells, and the demonstrated effect of AR inhibition on sorbitol and dulcitol production have long been documented [7–11]. We now propose an extremely active polyol removal in the human lens.

Acknowledgments

This project was supported by EY04424 from the National Eye Institute, National Institutes of Health. NMR studies were conducted at Massachusetts General Hospital NMR-Center, Charlestown, Mass., USA.

References

1 Cheng H-M: Nuclear magnetic resonance studies of ocular tissues. Med Sci Res 1988;15:441–446.
2 González RG, Miglior S, von Saltza I, Buckley L, Neuringer LJ, Cheng H-M: ^{31}P NMR studies of the diabetic lens. Magn Reson Med 1988;6:435–444.
3 Cheng H-M, Xiong H, Xiong J, Tsubota K: Metabolic studies of galactosemic cataract. Exp Eye Res 1990;51:345–349.
4 Cheng H-M, Xiong J, Tanaka G, Chang C, Asterlin AA, Aguayo JB: Analysis of concurrent glucose consumption by the hexose monophosphate shunt, glycolysis, and the polyol pathway in the crystalline lens. Exp Eye Res 1991;53:363–366.
5 Cheng H-M, Cheng FY, Xiong H, Xiong J: The further metabolism of sorbitol-3-phosphate and fructose-3-phosphate in the mature rat lens. Ophthalmic Res 1996;28:57–63.
6 Cheng H-M, González RG: Phosphorus-31 profiles of normal and diabetic human lenses. Med Sci Res 1991;19:91–92.
7 Robison WG Jr, Houlder N, Kinoshita JH: The role of lens epithelium in sugar cataract formation. Exp Eye Res 1990;50:641–646.
8 Chylack LT Jr, Henriquez HF III, Cheng H-M, Tung WH: Efficacy of Alrestatin, an aldose reductase inhibitor in human diabetic and non-diabetic lenses. Ophthalmology 1979;86:1579–1585.
9 Jedziniak JA, Chylack LT Jr, Cheng H-M, Gillis MK, Kalustian AA, Tung WH: The sorbitol pathway in the human lens: Aldose reductase and polyol dehydrogenase. Invest Ophthalmol Vis Sci 1981;20:314–326.
10 Lin LR, Reddy VN, Giblin FJ, Kador PF, Kinoshita JH: Polyol accumulation in cultured human epithelial cells. Exp Eye Res 1991;52:93–100.
11 Reddy VN, Lin LR, Giblin FJ, Lou M, Kador PF, Kinoshita JH: The efficacy of aldose reductase inhibitors on polyol accumulation in human lens and retinal pigment epithelium in tissue culture. J Ocul Pharmacol 1992;8:43–52.

Ophthalmic Research

Ophthalmic Res 1996;28(suppl 2):11–15

Shuji Matsukura
Masayasu Bando
Hajime Obazawa

Department of Ophthalmology, Tokai University School of Medicine, Isehara, Kanagawa, Japan

Ferricyanide Reductase Activity in Cataractous Human Lens

Key Words
Cataractous human lens
Ferricyanide reductase activity
Soluble fraction
Insoluble fraction
Lens protein aggregation

Abstract
We assayed ferricyanide reductase activity (one of NADH-dependent diaphorase activities) in the soluble and insoluble fractions of cataractous human lenses. Activity of this reductase in both the soluble and insoluble fractions tended to decrease in order of cortex > nucleus periphery > nucleus center, and it was suggested that a decrease of the reductase activity is closely correlated with lens protein aggregation, and to some extent associated with the development of nuclear sclerosis (coloration) and cortical cataract. Furthermore, insoluble fraction had very high specific activity per mg insoluble protein in cortex, and the activity decreased sharply with an increase in the level of insoluble protein. The reductase activity in the insoluble fraction may be also related to the metabolic activity of plasma membranes.

Introduction

Oxidation of the lens constituents is early event in the development of senile cataract, and lens protein aggregates are formed by oxidation [1]. Such oxidation may be associated with a decrease in the reducing activities of the lens. The lens is usually maintained in a high reduction state, and protected from oxidative stress by the antioxidation mechanisms such as the glutathione [2], ascorbate [3] and diaphorase (NAD(P)H-dependent reductase of xenobiotic compounds) [4] redox systems.

Recently, we [5] have found that ferricyanide reductase activity (one of diaphorase activities) is widely distributed in the soluble and granular (plasma membrane) fractions in

KARGER

E-Mail karger@karger.ch
Fax + 41 61 306 12 34
http://www.karger.ch

© 1996 S. Karger AG, Basel
0030–3747/96/0288–0011$10.00/0

Shuji Matsukura, MD
Department of Ophthalmology
Tokai University School of Medicine
Isehara, Kanagawa 259-11 (Japan)

Table 1. Ferricyanide reductase activities per mg tissue protein in the soluble and insoluble fractions of cataractous human lens cortex

% insoluble protein	Ferricyanide reductase activity nmol NADH oxidized/min/mg tissue protein			Cortical opacity
	soluble fraction	insoluble fraction	total	
2.9	64.4	7.4	71.8	–
6.4	42.7	27.2	69.9	2+
9.8	25.3	16.8	42.1	1+
12.1	29.8	23.6	53.4	–
12.8	40.5	45.1	85.6	1+
21.4	16.3	8.4	24.7	3+
28.8	36.2	14.9	51.1	2+
68.7	42.6	0	42.6	3+*

* Morgagnian mature cataract. – = The absence of cortical opacity.

the human lens, and suggested that its activity may play some role in keeping the lens reduction state. The diaphorase activity is specific for NADH, and its activity in the granular fractions is presumably bound to the plasma membranes since the granular activity was increased by treatment with 1% Triton X-100 [6].

The present study was undertaken to examine the relationship of ferricyanide reductase activity in the soluble and insoluble fractions of cataractous human lens cortex and nucleus to lens protein aggregation, lens opacity and nuclear sclerosis.

Materials and Methods

Eight cortices and 9 nucleuses of cataractous human lenses were obtained from 17 patients of 49–87 years old by extracapsular cataract extraction surgery in the operating rooms of the Ophthalmology Departments of the Tokai University Hospital and Isehara Kyodo Hospital. Lens cortex obtained was a small part of the whole cortex; cortical remnants (a part of equatorial and posterior cortex) after the delivery of lens nucleus or a part of anterior cortex collected before the lens nucleus delivery. One transparent whole lens (56 years old) was also obtained by intracapsular lens extraction because of traumatic lens dislocation. Each lens sample was kept frozen at –80 °C until used within about 1 week. Preoperatively, the cataractous and transparent lenses were examined by slit lamp biomicroscopy, and in this study, the grade of cortical cataract and nuclear sclerosis were described. The grade of cortical opacity was divided into three stages; 1+ to mature cataract of 3+, but the grades estimated as 1+ and 2+ might or might not coincide with the turbidity grades of the obtained cortical samples which should not represent the whole lenses. Nuclear sclerosis was classified into 1+ to 3+ based on color.

The nucleus of cataractous lenses was dissected into easily crushable peripheral and hard central parts. The transparent lens was also dissected out until the hard inner portion emerged, and the crushed outer portion and the remaining inner portion were considered to be nucleus periphery (including cortex and capsule epithelium) and nucleus center, respectively. Each cortex, nucleus periphery or nucleus center was homogenized in ice-cold 50 m*M* K-phosphate, pH 7.2 at a protein concentration of less than 10 mg/ml using a glass homogenizer, and then the soluble and insoluble fractions in homogenate were separated by centrifugation at 22,000 *g* for 30 min at 4 °C. Ferricyanide reductase activity in the lens soluble and insoluble fractions was spectrophotometrically determined in 1% Triton X-100, 50 m*M* K-phosphate buffer at 27 °C by measuring the oxidation rate of 100 μ*M* NADH at 340 nm in the presence of 150 μ*M* ferricyanide, as described previously [6, 7]. Protein was assayed by the BCA method [8] using bovine serum albumin as the standard.

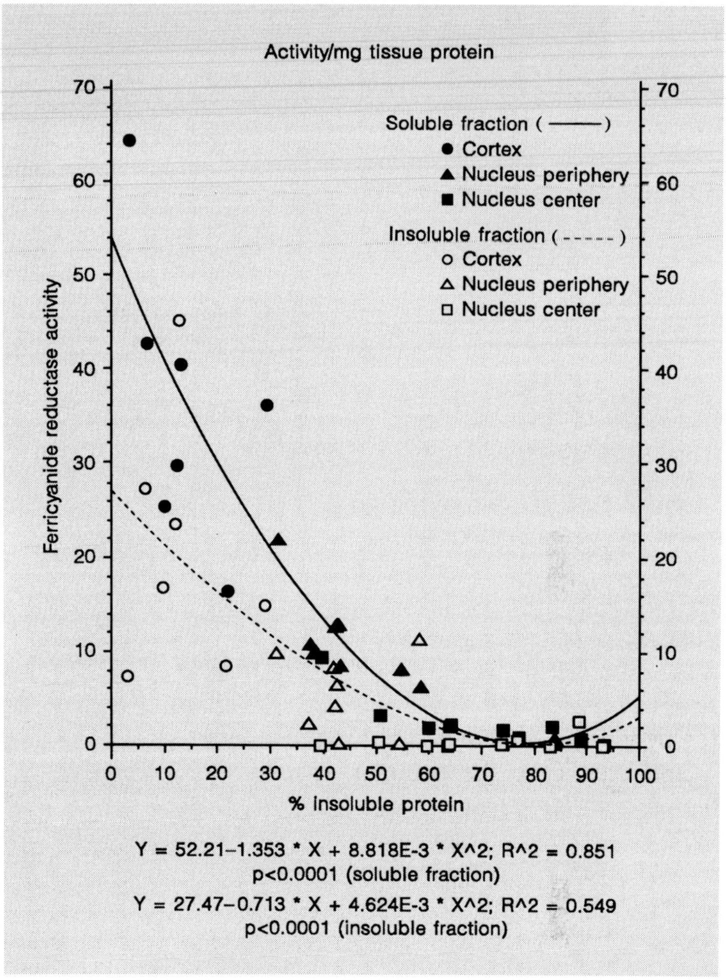

Fig. 1. Plots of ferricyanide reductase activities per mg tissue protein in the soluble and insoluble fractions of cortex and nucleus of cataractous human lenses against their % insoluble protein. The data of a Morgagnian mature cataract, as shown in table 1, were excluded from this figure because of the reason described in the text. Regression analysis: for the soluble fraction (—), $Y = 52.21 - 1.353X + 0.008818X^2$ ($R^2 = 0.851$, $p < 0.0001$); for the insoluble fraction (---), $Y = 27.47 - 0.713X + 0.004624X^2$ ($R^2 = 0.549$, $p < 0.0001$).

Results and Discussion

Table 1 shows ferricyanide reductase activities per mg tissue protein in the soluble and insoluble fractions of cataractous human lens cortex. The activities are tabulated according to low to high % insoluble protein which is expressed as percent of total protein content. Two mature cataracts exhibit the lowest activity in either the soluble or insoluble fraction of cortex. In cortex of a Morgagnian mature cataract, however, an abnormal high proportion of insoluble protein and high activity of the soluble reductase are observed, and this apparent observation may be caused by proteolyzing and leakage of a lot of soluble protein in the cataract. Figure 1 depicts clearly that the reductase activity in both the soluble and insoluble fractions tends to decrease in order of cortex > nucleus periphery > nucleus center, and to decrease with the increase of % insoluble protein. One peripheral and two central samples of two analyzed nucleuses with the hardest sclerosis of 3+ contained

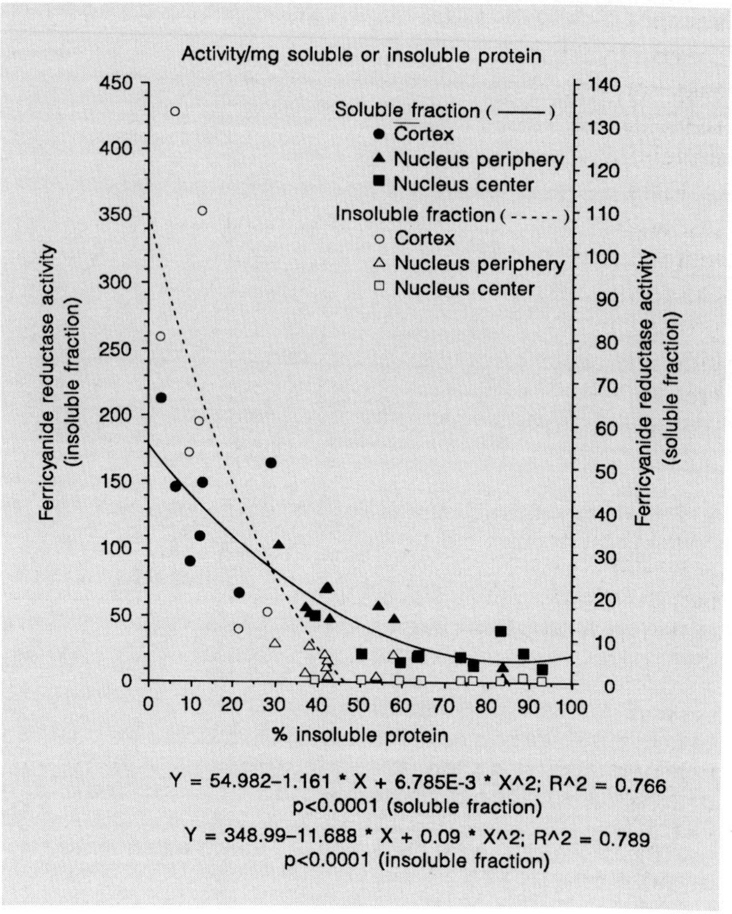

Fig. 2. Plots of ferricyanide reductase activities per mg soluble or insoluble protein in each fraction of cortex and nucleus of cataractous human lenses against their % insoluble protein. The data of a Morgagnian mature cataract were exluded from this figure as well as figure 1. Regression analysis: for the soluble fraction (—), $Y = 54.982 - 1.161X + 0.006785X^2$ ($R^2 = 0.766$, $p < 0.0001$); for the insoluble fraction (---), $Y = 348.99 - 11.688X + 0.09X^2$ ($R^2 = 0.789$, $p < 0.0001$).

more than 80% insoluble protein, and exhibited the lowest activity level, whereas the nuclear sclerosis of 1+ or 2+ was found in the nuclear samples with some higher activity levels in a wide region of about 40–80% insoluble protein.

From the above results, it is suggested that a decrease in the lens ferricyanide reductase activity is closely correlated with lens protein aggregation, and to some extent associated with the development of nuclear sclerosis (coloration) and cortical cataract. Previous papers [3, 9] have reported that a similar correlation between the activity decline and lens protein aggregation is also observed in the lens ascorbate free radical (AFR) reductase activity, 70–90% of which is found in the soluble fraction. Our recent chromatographic and enzymological investigation [10] indicates that about half and half of ferricyanide reductase activity in the lens soluble fraction may originate from AFR reductase and NADH-cytochrome b_5 reductase. NADH-cytochrome b_5 reductase is known to be widely distributed in the microsome and cytosol of various tissues [11], and to catalyze the one-electron reduction of xenobiotic compounds [12]. AFR reductase is a key enzyme of the ascorbate redox system [3], and possesses diaphorase activity as well [7, 10]. In the human lens, thus, it is suggested that the enzymes with ferricyanide reductase activity may protect structural lens proteins against various oxidants.

Figure 2 shows plots of ferricyanide reductase activities per mg soluble or insoluble protein in each fraction of cortex and nucleus of cataractous lenses against their % insoluble protein. Insoluble fraction has very high specific activity in cortex, and the activity decreases sharply with an increase of % insoluble protein. This result suggests that the reductase may be localized in a much higher activity on the metabolically active plasma membranes of cortex. It has been described that redox systems in plasma membranes may be related to several vital functions of cells [13]. The apparent K_m values of ferricyanide reductase activity in the lens insoluble fraction for NADH and ferricyanide are similar to those of NADH-cytochrome b_5 reductase [6]. However, a few enzymes in plasma membranes exhibit ferricyanide reductase activity [13]. Therefore, a further chromatographic and enzymological investigation is necessary to elucidate the molecular properties of the reductase activity in the lens-insoluble fraction in conjunction with researching its vital function(s).

Acknowledgments

This investigation was supported in part by a joint research project from the Eye Research Institute of the Cataract Foundation, Tokyo, Japan, and a research grant from the Welfare Ministry of Japan. We thank Dr. Kenji Ito of the Isehara Kyodo Hospital for providing us with cataractous human lenses.

References

1 Spector A: Oxidation and cataract; in Nugent J, Whelan J (eds): Human Cataract Formation, Ciba Found Symp 106. London, Pitman, 1984, pp 48–64.
2 Reddy VN, Giblin FJ: Metabolism and function of glutathione in the lens; in Nugent J, Whelan J (eds): Human Cataract Formation. Ciba Found Symp 106. London, Pitman, 1984, pp 65–87.
3 Bando M, Obazawa H: Activities of ascorbate free radical reductase and H_2O_2-dependent NADH oxidation in senile cataractous human lenses. Exp Eye Res 1990;50:779–784.
4 Tumminia SJ, Rao PV, Zigler JS Jr, Russell P: Xenobiotic induction of quinone oxidoreductase activity in lens epithelial cells. Biochim Biophys Acta 1993;1203:251–259.
5 Bando M, Obazawa H, Ishii Y: Reduced nicotinamide adenine dinucleotide-dependent reductase in the human lens. Atarashii Ganka (J Eye) 1993;10:483–487.
6 Bando M, Matsukura S, Obazawa H: Ferricyanide reductase activity in the soluble and plasma membrane fractions of the human lens. Atarashii Ganka (J Eye) 1994;11: 1124–1126.
7 Bando M, Obazawa H: Soluble ascorbate free radical reductase in the human lens. Jpn J Ophthalmol 1994;38:1–9.
8 Smith PK, Krohn RI, Hermanson GT, Mallia AK, Gartner FH, Provenzano MD, Fujimoto EK, Goeke NM, Olson BJ, Klenk DC: Measurement of protein using bicinchoninic acid. Anal Biochem 1985;150:76–85.
9 Bando M, Obazawa H: Regional and subcellular distribution of ascorbate free radical reductase activity in the human lens. Tokai J Exp Clin Med 1991;16:217–222.
10 Bando M, Obazawa H: Ascorbate free radical reductases and diaphorases in soluble fractions of the human lens. Tokai J Exp Clin Med 1995;20:in press.
11 Leroux A, Junien C, Kaplan J-C, Bamberger J: Generalised deficiency of cytochrome b_5 reductase in congenital methaemoglobinaemia with mental retardation. Nature 1975;258:619–620.
12 Iyanagi T, Yamazaki I: One-electron-transfer reactions in biochemical systems. III. One-electron reduction of quinones by microsomal flavin enzymes. Biochim Biophys Acta 1969;172:370–381.
13 Crane FL, Sun IL, Clark MG, Grebing C, Löw H: Transplasma-membrane redox systems in growth and development. Biochim Biophys Acta 1985;811:233–264.

Ophthalmic Research

Ophthalmic Res 1996;28(suppl 2):16–25

Yoshiji Ohta[a]
Hiroshi Okada[b]
Yoshinao Majima[b]
Isao Ishiguro[a]

Departments of
[a] Biochemistry and
[b] Ophthalmology, School of Medicine, Fujita Health University, Toyoake, Aichi, Japan

Anticataract Action of Vitamin E: Its Estimation Using an in vitro Steroid Cataract Model

Key Words
Methylprednisolone
Steroid cataract
Vitamin E
Oxidative damage
Membrane dysfunction
Cultured rat lens

Abstract
The aim of this study was to estimate the anticataract action of vitamin E using an in vitro methylprednisolone (MP)-induced cataract model. The same severity of early cortical cataract was induced in lenses isolated from male Wistar rats aged 6 weeks by incubation with MP (1.5 mg/ml) in TC-199 medium. The cataractous lenses showed slight increases in lipid peroxide (LPO) content and Na^+/K^+ ratio and slight decreases in reduced glutathione (GSH) content and glyceraldehyde-3-phosphate dehydrogenase (GAP-DH), a sensitive index of oxidative stress, and Na^+,K^+-ATPase activities. When the cataractous lenses were further incubated in TC-199 medium with and without vitamin E (250 μg/ml) for 48 h, the progression of cataract was prevented in the vitamin E-treated lenses, but not in the vitamin E-untreated lenses. The vitamin E-untreated lenses showed a decrease in vitamin E content and an increase in water content in addition to further increases in LPO content and Na^+/K^+ ratio and further decreases in GSH content and GAP-DH and Na^+,K^+-ATPase activities. In contrast, the changes of these components and enzymes except for GSH were attenuated in the vitamin E-treated lenses. From these results, it can be estimated that vitamin E prevents in vitro cataractogenesis in rat lenses treated with MP by protecting the lenses against oxidative damage and loss of membrane function.

KARGER

E-Mail karger@karger.ch
Fax + 41 61 306 12 34
http://www.karger.ch

© 1996 S. Karger AG, Basel
0030–3747/96/0288–0016$10.00/0

Yoshiji Ohta, PhD
Department of Biochemistry
School of Medicine
Fujita Health University
Toyoake, Aichi 470-11 (Japan)

Introduction

It has been demonstrated that vitamin E prevents cataractogenesis in a variety of in vivo and in vitro cataract models [1–3]. Creighton et al. [4] have reported that vitamin E partially prevents opacification of rat lenses cultured with methylprednisolone (MP). Recently, we have shown that vitamin E content decreases with an increase in lipid peroxide (LPO) content and decreases in reduced glutathione (GSH) content and glyceraldehyde-3-phosphate dehydrogenase (GAP-DH) activity at the late stage of cataractogenesis in cultured rat lenses with MP treatment [5]. In addition, we have reported that vitamin E can prevent cataract progression in rat lenses cultured with MP when the vitamin treatment is conducted at the early stage of the cataractogenesis, but not at the late stage [6]. However, it is not still enough to estimate the preventive action of vitamin E on this in vitro cataractogenesis in MP-treated rat lenses.

We, therefore, attempted to estimate the anti-cataract action of vitamin E using this in vitro MP-induced cataract model. Namely, we examined the preventive effect of vitamin E on cataract progression and changes of vitamin E, LPO, GSH, and water contents, Na^+/K^+ ratio, and GAP-DH, which is known to be sensitive to oxidative stress [7], and Na^+/K^+-ATPase activities in rat lenses with early cortical cataract induced by MP treatment following further incubation in a culture medium containing MP. Vitamin E is well known to function not only as a chain-breaking antioxidant but also as a membrane stabilizer [8, 9]. Mayman et al. [10] have reported using bovine lenses cultured with dexamethasone that the dysfunction of the cation pump via Na^+,K^+-ATPase might be related to cataractogenesis. Accordingly, Na^+/K^+ ratio, water content, and Na^+/K^+-ATPase activity in lenses were checked to estimate the membrane function in addition to the determinations of vitamin E, LPO, and GSH contents and GAP-DH activity in the tissues.

Materials and Methods

Chemicals

MP (6α-methylprednisolone 21-hemi-succinate) was purchased from Sigma Chemical Co. (St. Louis, Mo., USA); powder TC-199 and fetal calf serum (FCS) from Gibco Laboratories Life Technologies Inc. (Grand Island, N.Y., USA); a mixture of antibiotics (penicillin, streptomycin, and fungisone) from Bio-Whittaker (Walkersville, Mass., USA); vitamin E dissolved in HCO-60 and HCO-60 from Esai Co. (Tokyo, Japan); ATP, 3-phosphoglycerate, and 3-phosphoglycerate kinase from Boehringer Mannheim (Tokyo, Japan). Other chemicals used were commercially available and of reagent grade.

Animals

Male Wistar rats aged 6 weeks were used throughout. The animals were purchased from SLC Co. (Hamamatsu, Japan). All animals received human care in compliance with the institution's guidelines.

Isolation and Culture of Lenses

Eyes were enucleated from rats immediately after sacrifice by cervical dislocation. Lenses were dissected from the eyes using the posterior approach. Each isolated lens was placed in one well of a Falcon plastic culture plate (24 wells) (Becton Dickinson Labware, Franklin Lakes, N.J., USA) which contained 2 ml of a culture medium consisting of TC-199/bicarbonate buffer (pH 7.4), 10% FCS, 0.1 ml of a mixed solution of antibiotics, and 5.6 m*M* glucose (basic medium). They were incubated at 37 °C under 90% moisture and 95% air-5% CO_2 gas atmosphere for 24 h. A transient increase in lens wet weight was observed during this incubation as described in our previous report [11], but the incubated lenses showed the same wet weight as fresh lenses dissected from the eyes. Then, each of the resulting transparent lenses was incubated in 2 ml of the basic culture medium containing MP (1.5 mg/ml) for 24 h to induce early cataracts around the cortical equator or in 2 ml of the basic medium for the same period as the control. Next, each of the MP-treated lenses with the same severity of cortical opacity was incubated in 2 ml of the basic medium containing MP (1.5 mg/ml) with and without vitamin E (250 μg/ml) for 24 and 48 h, while each of the MP-untreated clear

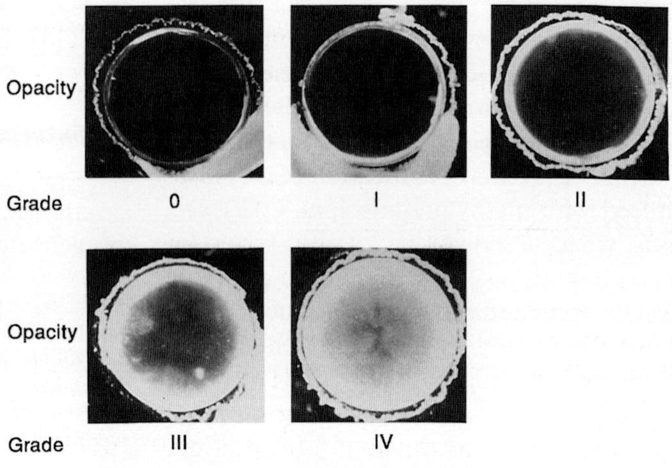

Fig. 1. Gradation of opacity in rat lenses cultured with MP. Grade 0 = No opacity; grade I = faint cortical opacity around the equator: grade II = cortical opacity slightly spreading from the equator toward the center part of lens; grade III = cortical opacity spreading nearby the center part of lens; grade IV = cortical opacity covering the whole part of lens.

lenses was incubated in 2 ml of the basic medium with and without vitamin E (250 μg/ml) for the same period. During these incubations, PM-untreated clear lenses showed no significant change in wet weight. The volume of a vitamin E solution in HCO-60, a detergent, added to the medium was 10 μl. When lenses with and without MP treatment were not incubated with vitamin E, 10 μl of a HCO-60 solution used for dissolution of vitamin E was added to the medium. Immediately after observation of opacity, lenses were lightly blotted on a filter, weighed, and then kept in a small plastic tube with a tight cap which was filled with nitrogen gas at –80 °C until use.

Estimation of the Severity of Lens Opacity

Lens opacity was checked by the dark field photographic method described in our previous reports [5, 6, 11], using a dissecting microscope, Olympus SHZ-ILL, equipped with an automatic microscope camera, Olympus PM-10AD (Olympus Optical Co., Tokyo, Japan). The severity of lens opacity was estimated based on the opacity gradation as shown in figure 1.

Measurements of Vitamin E, GSH, LPO, and Water in Lenses

Vitamin E in lenses was measured by the method of Abe et al. [12] using high-performance liquid chromatography with fluorescence detection. The amount of vitamin E measured is expressed as that of α-tocopherol (α-Toc). GSH in lenses was measured by the method of Sedlak and Lindsay [13] using Ellman's reagent. LPO in lenses was measured according to the method of Ohkawa et al. [14] using 2-thiobarbituric acid reactione except that 1.0 m*M* ethylenediaminetetraacetic acid was added to the reaction mixture. The amount of LPO measured is expressed as that of malondialdehyde (MDA). Water in lenses was determined as follows: Lenses were dried at 100 °C in an electric oven for 30 h after checking their wet weight and then their dry weight was checked again after cooling. Water content in lenses was estimated by subtracting their dry weight from their wet weight. This content is expressed as the percentage of water contained in lenses.

Measurement of Na^+/K^+ Ratio in Lenses

Na^+ and K^+ in lenses were determined using a Hitachi model 710 automatic electrolytes analyzer (Hitachi Co., Tokyo, Japan). Na^+/K^+ ratio in lenses was calculated based on the contents of Na^+ and K^+ in the tissues.

Assays of GAP-DH and Na^+,K^+-ATPase in Lenses

GAP-DH in lenses was assayed according to the method of Bergmeyer et al. [15]. The oxidation of NADH to NAD^+ following the conversion of 1,3-diphosphoglycerate to glyceraldehyde via the enzyme was measured in the reaction mixture consisting of 1.1 m*M* ATP, 6.2 m*M* 3-phosphoglycerate, 0.2 m*M* NADH, 0.9 m*M* ethylenediaminetetraacetic acid, 2.0 m*M* $MgCl_2$, 13 units of 3-phosphoglycerate kinase, and

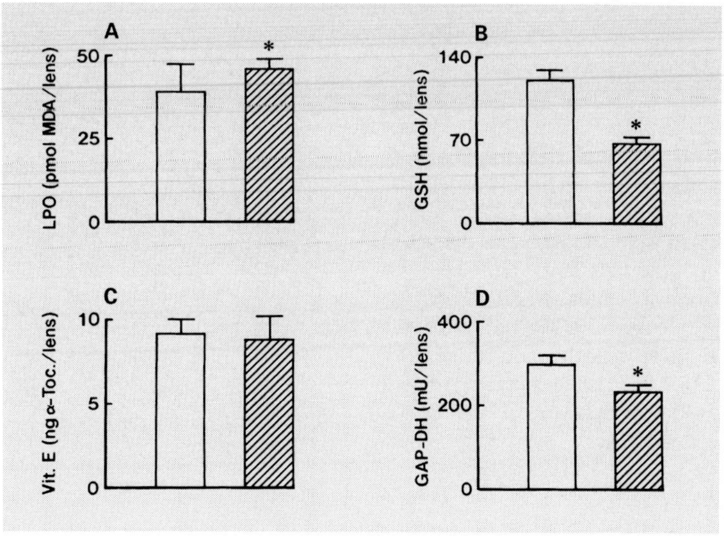

Fig. 2. LPO (**A**), GSH (**B**), and vitamin E (**C**) contents and GAP-DH activity (**D**) in rat lenses with MP-induced grade II opacity and without opacity. Treatment of lenses with MP and determinations of lenticular LPO, GSH, vitamin E, and GAP-DH indicated were conducted as described in 'Materials and Methods'. □ = Control lenses without opacity; ▨ = lenses with MP-induced grade II opacity. Each value is the mean ± SD from three experiments with 5–8 lenses each. * $p < 0.05$ (vs. control lenses).

an appropriate amount of 10% lens homogenates in 82.3 m*M* triethanolamine buffer (pH 7.6) (total volume, 1.0 ml) at 37 °C. The decrease in absorbance at 340 nm following the oxidation of NADH was measured for 4 min after starting the reaction. One unit (U) of this enzyme is expressed as the amount of enzyme to cause the oxidation of NADH at an initial rate of 1 μmol/min. The amount of NADH oxidized was calculated using an extinction coefficient of 6.22 $mM^{-1} \cdot cm^{-1}$ at 340 nm for NADH. Na^+,K^+-ATPase in lenses was assayed by the method of Nakao et al. [16]. This enzyme activity is expressed in terms of the amount of inorganic phosphorus (P_i) released from ATP hydrolyzed by the enzyme at 37 °C for the first 1 h incubation per lens. P_i was determined by the method of Goldenberg and Fernandez [17].

Statistical Analyses

Results obtained for lens components and enzymes are expressed as the means ± SD. The statistical analyses of these results were performed using the Student's t test. For results of the severity of lens opacity, statistical analyses were carried out using the Mann-Whitney test. Values of significance were set at $p < 0.05$ for both tests.

Results

Rat lenses with MP-induced early cortical cataract that were used throughout in this study had grade II opacity.

The contents of LPO, GSH, and vitamin E and the activity of GAP-DH were first examined in lenses with MP-induced grade II opacity. LPO content in the opaque lenses significantly increased and was 1.2-fold more than that in clear control lenses (fig. 2A). GSH content in the opaque lenses significantly decreased and was 56% of the control level (fig. 2B). There was no difference in vitamin E content between the opaque and clear control lenses (fig. 2C). GAP-DH activity in the opaque lenses significantly decreased and was 78% of the control level (fig. 2D).

Na^+/K^+ ratio, water content, and Na^+,K^+-ATPase activity were next examined in lenses with MP-induced grade II opacity. Na^+/K^+ ratio in the opaque lenses significantly increased and was 3.1-fold higher than that in clear control lenses (fig. 3A). There was no difference in water content between the opaque

Fig. 3. Na^+/K^+ ratio (**A**), water content (**B**), and Na^+,K^+-ATPase activity (**C**) in rat lenses with MP-induced grade II opacity and without opacity. Treatment of lenses with MP and determinations of lenticular Na^+/K^+ ratio, water content, and Na^+,K^+-ATPase indicated were conducted as described in 'Materials and Methods'. □ = Control lenses without opacity; ▨ = lenses with MP-induced grade II opacity. Each value is the mean ± SD from three experiments with 5–11 lenses each. * $p < 0.05$ (vs. control lenses).

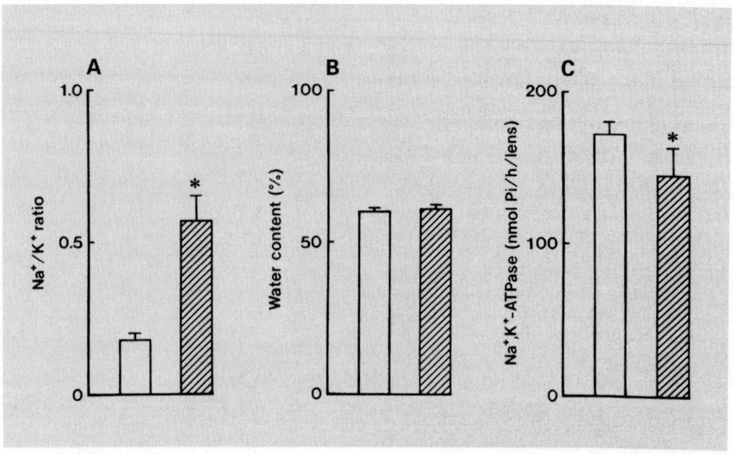

Fig. 4. Effect of vitamin E treatment on cataract progression in rat lenses with MP-induced grade II opacity following further incubation with MP for 24 and 48 h. Treatment of lenses with MP and vitamin E and estimation of cataract severity were conducted as described in 'Materials and Methods'. The number of lenses used is 30–31. * $p < 0.05$ (vs. vitamin E-untreated lenses).

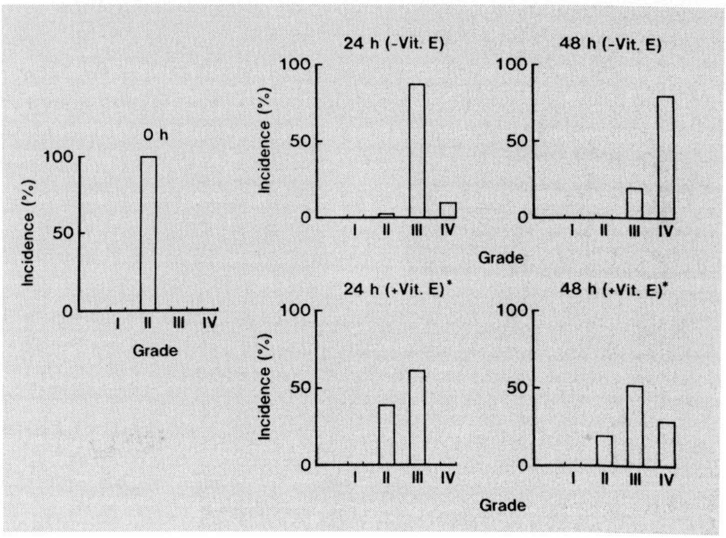

and clear control lenses (fig. 3B). Na^+,K^+-ATPase activity in the opaque lense significantly decreased and was 84% of the control level (fig. 3C).

When lenses with MP-induced grade II opacity were further incubated in a medium containing MP (1.5 mg/ml) with and without vitamin E (250 μg/ml) for 24 and 48 h, the progression of cataract occurred as shown in figure 4. In the lenses with grade II opacity which were incubated with MP in the absence of vitamin E for 24 h, incidence rates of grades II, III and IV opacity were 3, 87 and 10%, respectively. In contrast, incidence rates of grades II and III opacity were 39 and 61%, respectively, in the lenses with grade II opacity which were incubated with MP in the presence of vitamin E for 24 h. When the lenses with grade II opacity were incubated with MP in the absence of vitamin E for 48 h, grades III and IV opacity appeared at the rates of 20 and 80%, respectively. In contrast, grades II, III

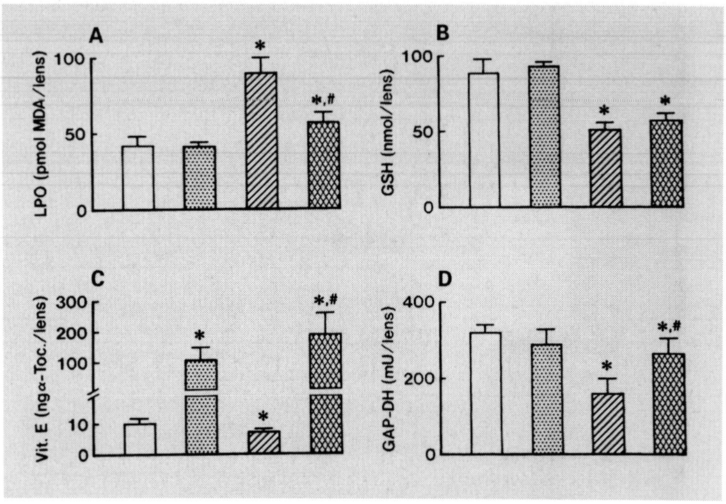

Fig. 5. Effect of vitamin E treatment on changes of LPO (**A**), GSH (**B**), and vitamin E (**C**) contents and GAP-DH activity (**D**) in rat lenses with MP-induced grade II opacity and without opacity following further incubation with and without MP for 48 h. Treatment of lenses with MP and/or vitamin E and determinations of lenticular LPO, GSH, vitamin E, and GAP-DH indicated were conducted as described in 'Materials and Methods'. □ = Control group (clear lenses with neither MP nor vitamin E treatments); ▩ = vitamin E-treated group (clear lenses with vitamin E treatment alone); ▨ = MP-treated group (opaque lenses with MP treatment alone); ▦ = MP + vitamine E-treated group (opaque lenses with MP and vitamin E treatments). Each value is a mean ± SD from three experiments with 4–5 lenses each. * $p < 0.05$ (vs. control group). # $p < 0.05$ (vs. MP-treated group).

and IV opacity appeared at the rates of 19, 52 and 29%, respectively, when the lenses with grade II opacity were incubated with MP in the presence of vitamin E for 48 h. Thus, vitamin E prevented the progression of MP-induced cataract and this preventive effect was significant.

When lenses with MP-induced grade II opacity were further incubated with MP (1.5 mg/ml) in the presence or absence of vitamin E (250 μg/ml) for 48 h, LPO, GSH, and vitamin E contents and GAP-DH activity in the tissues changed as shown in figure 5. The opaque lenses cultured with MP in the absence of vitamin E (MP-treated group) showed a significant increase in LPO content and significant decreases in GSH and vitamin E contents and GAP-DH activity. LPO content in the MP-treated group was 2.1-fold more than that in clear lenses cultured with neither MP nor vitamin E (control group) (fig. 5A). GSH content in the MP-treated group was 57% of that in the control group, while vitamin E content in the former group was 70% of that in the latter group (fig. 5B, C). GAP-DH activity in the MP-treated group was 50% of that in the control group (fig. 5D). LPO content in the opaque lenses cultured with MP in the presence of vitamin E (MP + vitamin E-treated group) was 1.3-fold more than that in the control group but was significantly less than that in the MP-treated group (fig. 5A). GSH content in the MP + vitamin E-treated group was 64% of that in the control group and this content was almost equivalent to that in the MP-treated group (fig. 5B). Vita-

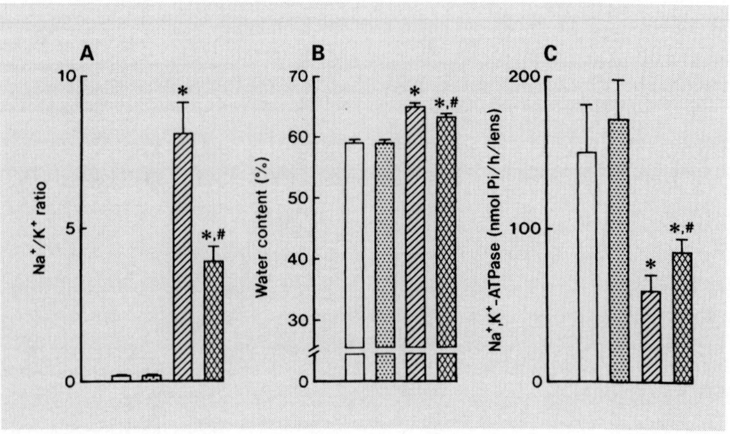

Fig. 6. Effect of vitamin E treatment on changes of Na^+/K^+ ratio (**A**), water content (**B**), and Na^+,K^+-ATPase activity (**C**) in rat lenses with MP-induced grade II opacity and without opacity following further incubation with and without MP for 48 h. Treatment of lenses with MP and/or vitamin E and determinations of lenticular Na^+/K^+ ratio, water content, and Na^+,K^+-ATPase indicated were conducted as described in 'Materials and Methods'. □ = Control group (clear lenses with neither MP nor vitamin E treatments); ▦ = vitamin E-treated group (clear lenses with vitamin E treatment alone); ▨ = MP-treated group (opaque lenses with MP treatment alone); ▩ = MP + vitamin E-treated group (opaque lenses with MP and vitamin E treatments). Each value is a mean ± SD from three experiments with 4–5 lenses each. * $p < 0.05$ (vs. control group). # $p < 0.05$ (vs. MP-treated group).

min E content in the MP + vitamin E-treated group was 20-fold more than that in the control group and was significantly higher than that in the MP-treated group (fig. 5C). GAP-DH activity in the MP + vitamin E-treated group was 83% of that in the control group but was significantly higher than that in the MP-treated group (fig. 5D). There were no significant changes in LPO and GSH contents and GAP-DH activity in clear lenses incubated with vitamin E (250 μg/ml) in the absence of MP for 48 h (vitamin E-treated group) (fig. 5A–C). Vitamin E content in the vitamin E-treated group was 11-fold more than that in the control group and was not significantly different from that in the MP + vitamin E-treated group (fig. 5C).

When lenses with MP-induced grade II opacity were further incubated with MP (1.5 mg/ml) in the presence or absence of vitamin E (250 μg/ml) for 48 h, Na^+/K^+ ratio, water content, Na^+,K^+-ATPase activity in the tissues changed as shown in figure 6. The opaque lenses cultured with MP in the absence of vitamin E (MP-treated group) showed significant increases in Na^+/K^+ ratio and water content and a significant decrease in Na^+,K^+-ATPase activity. Na^+/K^+ ratio in the MP-treated group was 40-fold higher than that in clear lenses cultured with neither MP nor vitamin E (control group) (fig. 6A). Water content in the MP-treated group was 1.12-fold more than that in the control group (fig. 6B). Na^+,K^+-ATPase activity in the MP-treated group was 39% of that in the control group (fig. 6C). Na^+/K^+ ratio in the opaque lenses cultured with MP in the presence of vitamin E (MP + vitamin E-treated group) was 19-fold higher than that in the control group but was significantly lower than that in the MP-treated group (fig. 6A). Water content in the vitamin E-treated group was significantly more than that in the control group but was significantly less than that in the MP + vitamin E-treated group (fig. 6B). Na^+,K^+-ATPase activity in the vitamin E-treated group was 57% of that in the control group but was significantly higher than that in the MP + vitamin E-treated group (fig. 6C). No significant changes in Na^+/K^+ ratio, water content, and Na^+,K^+-ATPase activity occurred in clear lenses incubated with vitamin E (250 μg/ml) in the absence of MP for 48 h (vitamin E-treated group) (fig. 6A–C).

Discussion

The present study was undertaken to estimate the anticataract action of vitamin E on cataractogenesis in rat lenses cultured with MP. In this study, we examined the effect of vitamin E on the progression of cataract and changes in not only vitamin E, GSH, and LPO contents and GAP-DH activity, which are indices of oxidative stress, but also Na^+/K^+ ratio, water content, and Na^+,K^+-ATPase activity, which are indices of membrane function, in rat lenses with MP-induced early cortical cataract following further MP treatment.

Increases in LPO content and Na^+/K^+ ratio and decreases in GSH content and Na^+,K^+-ATPase activity were found in rat lenses with MP-induced early cortical cataract, indicating the occurrence of oxidative damage and membrane dysfunction with increased membrane permeability in the cataractous lenses. When such cataractous lenses with oxidative damage and membrane dysfunction were further cultured in a medium containing MP over a 48-hour period, cataract progressed and consequently the whole cortex was covered with opacity. In the lenses with such advanced cortical cataracts, oxidative damage was aggravated with a decrease in vitamin E content and an increase in water content occurred with further loss of the membrane function with markedly increased membrane permeability. We have already reported that vitamin E content decreases with an increase in LPO content and decreases in GSH content and GAP-DH activity at the late stage of cataractogenesis in cultured rat lenses with MP treatment [5]. Accordingly, these results indicate that not only oxidative damage but also membrane dysfunction should be linked to the progression of cataract in rat lenses cultured with MP. These results also support the mechanism by which damage of the cation pump in the lens membrane takes part in in vitro cataractogenesis induced by corticosteroids, which has been proposed by Mayman et al. [10].

We have reported that vitamin E can prevent cataract progression in rat lenses cultured with MP when the vitamin treatment is conducted at the early stage of the cataractogenesis [6]. Vitamin E is well known to function as a chain-breaking antioxidant and a membrane stabilizer [8, 9]. It is known that Na^+,K^+-ATPase, a component of the cation pump mechanism, in lens membranes requires lipids and sulfhydryl (-SH) group for expression of its enzymatic activity, and that this enzyme in lens is inactivated by changes of membrane lipid composition and membrane fluidity in the tissue and by oxidation of -SH group in the enzyme protein [18–21]. Takenaka et al. [22] have demonstrated that vitamin E functions as an antioxidant on the oxidation of membrane protein thiols induced by free radicals generated in different sites. When rat lenses with MP-induced early cortical cataract were further incubated in a medium containing MP with vitamin E over a 48-hour period, the progression of cataract was found to be prevented significantly. In addition, this vitamin E treatment was found to depress increases in LPO and water content and Na^+/K^+ ratio and decreases in vitamin E content and GAP-DH and Na^+,K^+-ATPase activities in rat lenses with MP-induced early cataract following further incubation with MP. From these results, it is further defined that vitamin E is capable of preventing cataract progression in cultured rat lenses with MP-induced early cortical cataract following further MP treatment. These results also suggest that vitamin E can prevent the progression of cataract in the opaque rat lenses further cultured with MP by protecting the lenses against oxidative damage and loss of the membrane function. However, vitamin E treatment could not depress a decrease in GSH content in rat lenses with MP-induced early cataract following further incubation with MP, while the vitamin treatment had a preventive effect on the increase of LPO content and the decreases of vitamin E content and GAP-DH activity in the cataractous lenses following further incubation with MP as described above. Although it is not clear at present why vitamin E cannot depress this decrease in lenticular GSH content following further MP treatment, the reason may be explained as follows: In rat lenses with MP-induced early cortical cataract, not only oxidative damage but also membrane dysfunction with increased membrane permeability occurred as mentioned above. It has been reported that a similar membrane dysfunction with increased membrane permeability takes place in rat lenses with early cortical cataract induced by treatment with high concentrations of sugars such as glucose, galactose, and xylose in vitro [23–25]. Lou et al. [26] have shown that in in vitro xylose-treated rat lenses with early cortical cataract, a decrease in lenticular GSH levels may be due to its loss through the osmotically damaged leaky membrane. In addition, we have reported that in rat lenses cultured with a high concentration of glucose or xylose, vitamin E in a liposomal form cannot arrest a decrease in GSH content with the development of cortical cataract, although the vitamin prevents an increase in LPO content in the tissues [11, 27]. From these findings, it can be presumed that the decrease of GSH content found in rat lenses with MP-induced early cortical cataract may be due to not only oxidative damage but also its loss through the osmotically damaged leaky membrane, and that in lenses cultured with MP, vitamin E treatment after early cataract formation is unable to prevent the loss of GSH through the once oxidatively and osmotically damaged leaky membrane, resulting in no prevention of the decrease of lenticular GSH content.

In conclusion, the present results indicate that in rat lenses cultured with MP, oxidative damage and membrane dysfunction in the tissues should be closely related to the progression of cataract, and that vitamin E is able to prevent this cataract progression when the vitamin treatment is conducted at the early stage of the cataractogenesis. In addition, the present results lead us to estimate that vitamin E can prevent in vitro cataractogenesis in MP-treated rat lenses by protecting the lenses against oxidative damage and loss of the membrane function.

References

1 Gerster H: Antioxidant vitamins in cataract prevention. Z Ernährungswiss 1989;28:56–75.

2 Machlin LJ: Influence of antioxidant vitamins on cataract formation; in Hayaishi O, Niki E, Kondo M, Yoshikawa T (eds): Medical, Biochemical and Clinical Aspects of Free Radicals. Amsterdam, Elsevier, 1989, pp 351–359.

3 Ohta Y, Ishiguro I: Causative factors of cataract and its prevention. Bio Industry 1995;12:13–24.

4 Creighton MO, Sanwal M, Stewart-DeHaan PJ, Trevithick JR: Modelling cortical cataractogenesis. 5. Steroid cataracts induced by solumedrol partially prevented by vitamin E in vitro. Exp Eye Res 1983;37:65–75.

5 Okada H, Ito A, Majima Y, Ohta Y, Ishiguro I, Torii H: Changes in vitamin E and related compounds in rat lenses cultured with methylprednisolone following opacification. J Eye (Atarashii Ganka) 1993;10:1263–1266.

6 Okada H, Majima Y, Ohta Y, Ishiguro I, Ito A, Torii H: Preventive effect of vitamin E on cataractogenesis in cultured rat lenses with steroid treatment. J Eye (Atarashii Ganka) 1994;11:79–83.

7 Spector A, Huang R-RC, Wang G-M, Schmidt C, Yan G-Z, Chifflet S: Dose elevated glutathione protect the cell from H_2O_2 insult? Exp Eye Res 1987;45:453–465.

8 Liebler DC: The role of metabolism in the antioxidant function of vitamin E. Clin Rev Toxicol 1993;23: 147–169.

9 Urano S: Membrane-stabilizing effect of vitamin E. Vitamins (Bitamin) 1989;63:75–85.

10 Mayman CI, Miller D, Tijerina ML: In vitro production of steroid cataract in bovine lens. 2. Measurement of sodium-potassium adenosine triphosphatase activity. Acta Ophthalmol 1979;57:1107–1116.

11 Ohta Y, Torri H, Okada H, Hattori H, Majima Y, Ishiguro I: Involvement of oxidative stress in *D*-xylose-induced cataractogenesis in cultured rat lenses. Curr Eye Res 1996;15:1–7.

12 Abe K, Yuguchi Y, Katsui G: Quantitative determination of tocopherols by high-speed liquid chromatography. J Nutr Sci Vitaminol 1975; 21:183–188.

13 Sedlak J, Lindsay RH: Estimation of total, protein-bound and nonprotein sulfhydryl groups in tissue with Ellman's reagent. Anal Biochem 1968; 25:192–205.

14 Ohkawa H, Ohishi N, Yagi K: Assay for lipid peroxides in animal tissues by thiobarbituric acid reaction. Anal Biochem 1979;95:351–358.

15 Bergmeyer HU, Grassl M, Walter G-E: Glyceraldehyde-3-phosphate dehydrogenase; in Bergmeyer HU (ed): Methods of Enzymatic Analysis. Weinheim, Verlag Chemie, 1983, vol II, pp 211–213.

16 Nakao T, Nagano K, Adachi K, Nakao M: Separation of two adenosine triphosphatases (ATPase) from erythrocyte membranes. Biochem Biophys Res Commun 1963;13: 444–448.

17 Goldenberg H, Fernandez A: Simplified method for the estimation of inorganic phosphate in body fluids. Clin Chem 1966;12:871–992.

18 Baghieri S, Garner MH: Na/K-ATPase and phospholipid degradation in bovine and human lenses. Curr Eye Res 1992;11:459–467.

19 Mizuno GR, Chapman CJ, Chipault JR, Pfeiffer DR: Lipid composition and (Na^+ + K^+)-ATPase activity in rat lens during triparanol-induced cataractogenesis. Biochim Biophys Acta 1981;644:1–12.

20 Sen PC, Pfeiffer DR: Characterization of partially purified (Na^+ + K^+)-ATPase from porcine lens. Biochim Biophys Acta 1982;693:34–44.

21 Fukui HN, Merola LO, Kinoshita JH: The effects of oxidants on the membrane sulfhydryl groups of the lens. Doc Ophthalmol 1976;8:161–169.

22 Takenaka Y, Miki M, Yasuda H, Mino M: The effect of α-tocopherol as an antioxidant on the oxidation of membrane protein thiols induced by free radicals generated in different sites. Arch Biochem Biophys 1991;285:344–350.

23 Kinoshita JH, Merola LO, Dikmak E: Osmotic changes in experimental galactose cataracts. Exp Eye Res 1962;1:405–410.

24 Obazawa H, Merola LO, Kinoshita JH: The effect of xylose on the isolated lens. Invest Ophthalmol 1974; 13:204–209.

25 Kinoshita JH: Mechanism initiating cataract formation. Proctor Lecture. Invest Ophthalmol 1974;13:713–724.

26 Lou MF, McKellar R, Chyan O: Quantitation of lens protein mixed disulfides by ion-exchange chromatography. Exp Eye Res 1986;42: 607–616.

27 Hattori H, Majima Y, Nagamura Y, Ishiguro I: Effect of vitamin E-containing liposome on experimental sugar cataract. Acta Soc Ophthalmol Jpn (Nippon Ganka Gakkai Zasshi) 1989;93:97–102.

Ophthalmic
Research

Ophthalmic Res 1996;28(suppl 2):26–31

Won Tae Jung[a]
Sae Hyun Rho[b]
Woo Chan Park[b]

[a] Department of Instrumental Analysis, Il Yang Central Research Institute, Kyungki;
[b] Department of Ophthalmology, Dong A University, Pusan, Korea

Racemization of Lens Crystalline Constituents in UV-Induced Cataract Evaluated by Chiral GC/MS Spectroscopy

Key Words
Racemization
Crystalline
Chiral separation
UV-B
Cataract
Gas chromatography-single quadrupole mass spectroscopy

Abstract
The racemization of amino acids is hypothesized to cause cataract by disrupting the crystalline's tertiary structure, which, in turn, alters the optical characteristics of the lens. To better understand the role of these modifications in cataractogenesis, the changes in stereoisomer ratio of amino acids from lens crystalline by UV-B-induced cataract in animal models were studied using chiral separation gas chromatography-single quadrupole mass spectroscopy. The anticataract action of a compound, {[1-(phenylmethyl)-1H-indazol-3-yl]oxy}acetic acid lysinate, was also evaluated by this method.

Introduction

Cataract, generally defined as a disturbance of lens transparency, is responsible for visual impairment in over 40 million people and blindness in over half of all blind individuals – 17 million worldwide [1]. The etiology of cataract is very diverse and there are many different forms of cataract. Therefore, the precise cause of cataract is unknown but it is likely that a multitude of factors can influence various aspects of lens metabolism leading to the development of light-scattering centers and opacity. Currently, a cataractous condition is surgically correctable but the problems and costs associated with the current treatment suggest that alternative methods be developed for treatment or prevention, if possible. However, new methods to prevent or reverse cataract formation cannot be derived until the mechanism responsible for cataract formation is understood at the molecular level. The lens proteins (crystallines) are susceptible to accumulating a variety of posttranslational modifications that are thought to cause cataracts by disrupting the crystalline's tertiary structure, which, in turn, alters the optical characteristics of the lens and eventually leads

KARGER

E-Mail karger@karger.ch
Fax +41 61 306 12 34
http://www.karger.ch

© 1996 S. Karger AG, Basel
0030–3747/96/0288–0026$10.00/0

Won Tae Jung
Department of Instrumental Analysis
Il Yang Central Research Institute
Hagal 182-4, Kiheung
Yongin, Kyungki 449-900 (Korea)

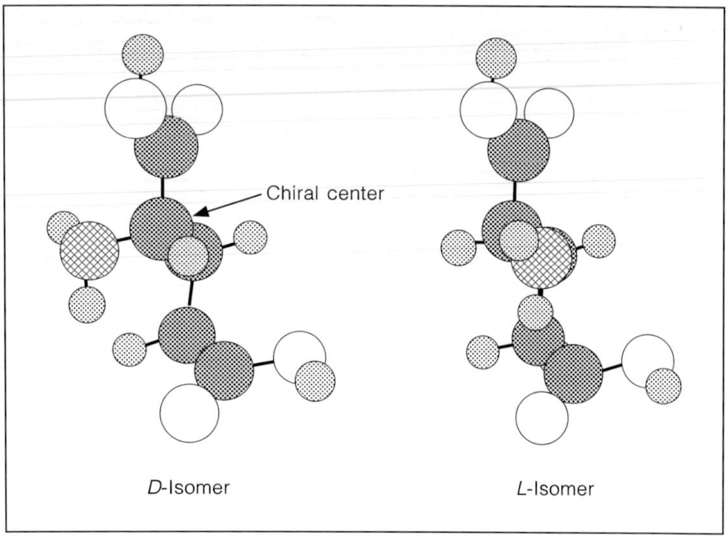

Fig. 1. Two enantiomers of an amino acid-glutamic acid.

to cataracts [2]. At the molecular level, these posttranslational modifications have been hypothesized to include nonenzymatic glycosylation of the free amino groups of lysine or the *N*-terminus, phosphorylation of serine, tyrosine or threonine residues, deamidation of glutamine and asparagine, truncation of the *C*-terminus, oxidation, cross-linking via disulfide bonds between cysteine residues, and cross-linking between glutamine; and lysyl residues catalyzed by transglutaminase [3–5].

Every amino acid except glycine has a chiral center and 2 enantiomers, as illustrated in figure 1.

Living cells have the unique ability to synthesize their *L*-amino acids only by stereospecific enzymes [6]. The optical isomers amino acids of crystalline very slowly undergo spontaneous nonenzymatic racemization to *D*-forms by aging or pathological process such as cataract [7]. To better understand the role of these modifications in cataractogenesis, e.g. UV-B-induced as a major factor of senile cataract, and to evaluate an anticataract compound – {[1-(phenylmethyl)-1H-indazol-3-yl]oxy} acetic acid lysinate (bendazac lysine) [8] – for its preventive action to cataract formation, we studied the changes in stereoisomer ratios from lens crystalline by UV-induced cataract using chiral capillary gas chromatography-mass spectroscopy. This study will show the methodology to evaluate the racemization of lens protein constituents-amino acids. The results elucidate that racemizations of crystalline amino acids have a strong possibility to change the tertiary structure of crystalline, which eventually causes lens opacity.

Materials and Methods

Animal Grouping and Treatment

The animals (all male, body weight 250 ± 20 g, age 2 months) were divided into 9 groups of 5 rats each. Eight groups (group/cage) except for the control were bred in a box shut off from exterior rays and exposed to 300–320 nm ultraviolet radiation (all day long, 0.1 mJ/cm^2) during 4–6 months either with or without administration of bendazac lysine. The administration of the compound was as follows: water-soluble lysine salt of bendazac 31.25 mg was dissolved in 150 ml of water and sup-

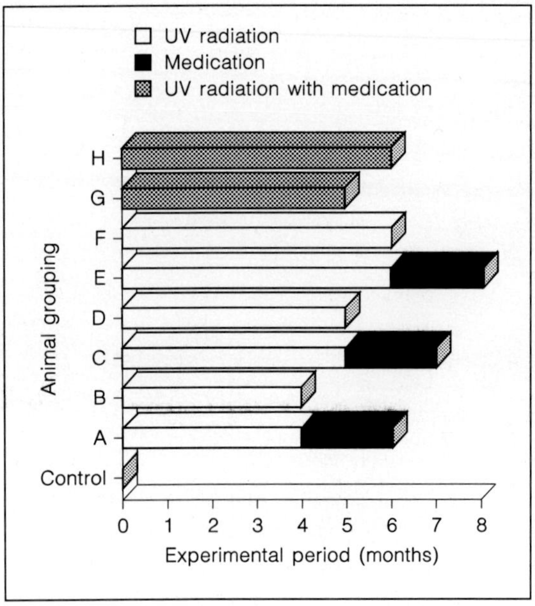

Fig. 2. Animal grouping and experimental treatment.

plied to 5 rats in a cage per day through a water bottle. The dosage to a rat was about 25 mg/kg/day p.o. To induce mydriasis 2–3 drops of 1% cyclopentolate solution was administered locally 3 times daily to each rat. After the treatment, UV-induced cataractous lenses were extracted and lyophilized for storage. The animal grouping, treatment and duration are shown in figure 2

Protein Fractionation from Lens

Proteins in lens were fractionated into water-soluble and -insoluble parts by Cotlier's method [9]. Polypeptide bonds of water-insoluble protein were broken down by hydrolysis.

Chiral Separation of Enantiomers

The hydrolyzed enatiomers were esterified as shown in figure 3.

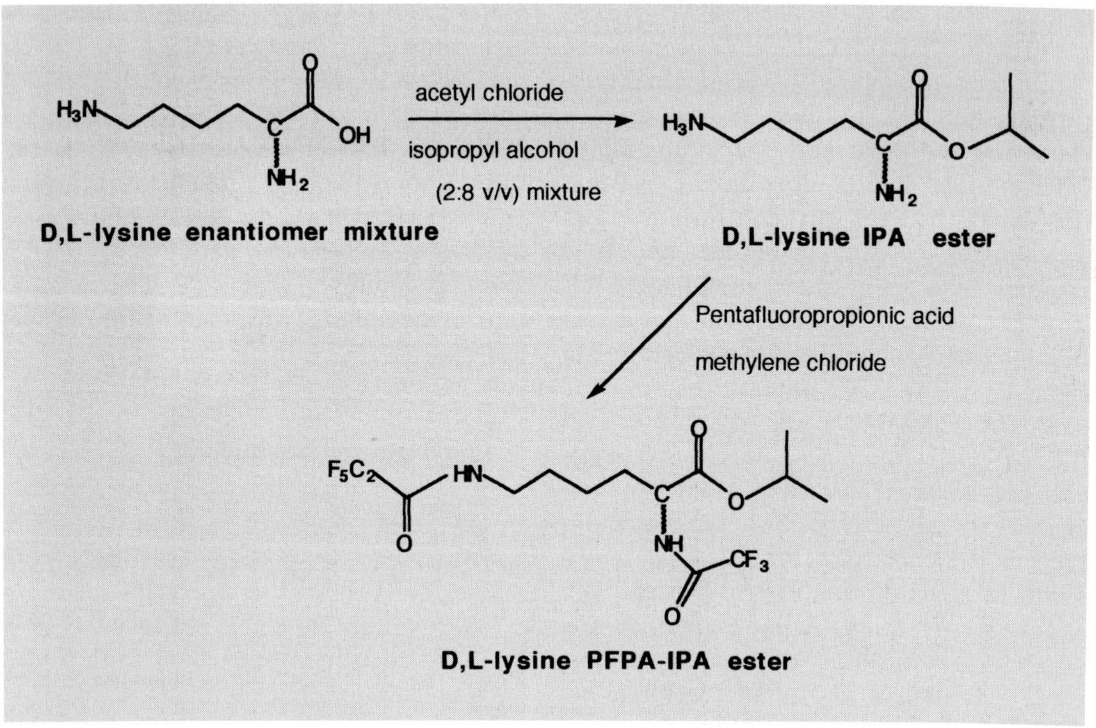

Fig. 3. Derivatization process of amino acid for chiral separation.

Then the enantiomers to be separated interact with the chiral stationary phase (*L*-valine *tert*-butyl-amide linked to polysiloxane) via hydrogen bonds to form diastereomeric association complexes with differences in their solvation enthalpy of a hundred calories [10]. Mass spectroscopy using quadrupole single-mass scan under conditions reported elsewhere [11] was carried out.

Results

Figure 4 shows the chromatography of *D,-L*-amino acids in water-insoluble protein from control lens. *D-,L*-Enantiomers of 10 amino acids were clearly separated. Some *D*-form enantiomers of serine, methionine, glutamic acid and lysine were found.

To confirm the chemical assignment of enantiomers, electron impact (EI)-mass spectra of enantiomers were obtained. Mass spectrum of glutamic acid for an example is shown in figure 5.

When the total dry weight of normal lenses is plotted against age after the first few years of rapid growth, an increase in apparent weight of approximately 0.4 mg/year has been found in human cases. Water-insoluble fraction increases at the same rate as the total dry weight. The water-soluble fraction remains constant at approximately 30 mg and the rate of conversion of soluble to insoluble material is constant in the normal lens. The *D/L* ratio of aspartic acid, for example, is constant at 0.036 in a water-soluble fraction, and the *D/L* ratio increases by 0.17%/year in a water-insoluble fraction. In cataract, the water-insoluble fraction increases dramatically due to a more

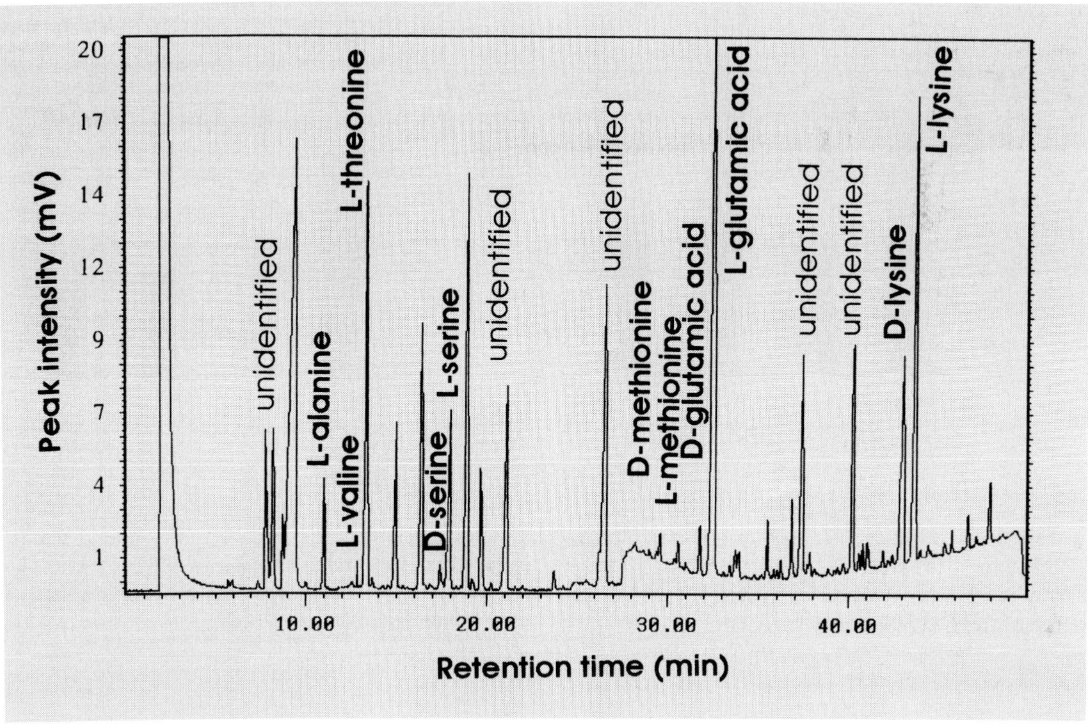

Fig. 4. Chromatogram of *D,L*-enantiomers of amino acids of the water-insoluble protein of control lenses.

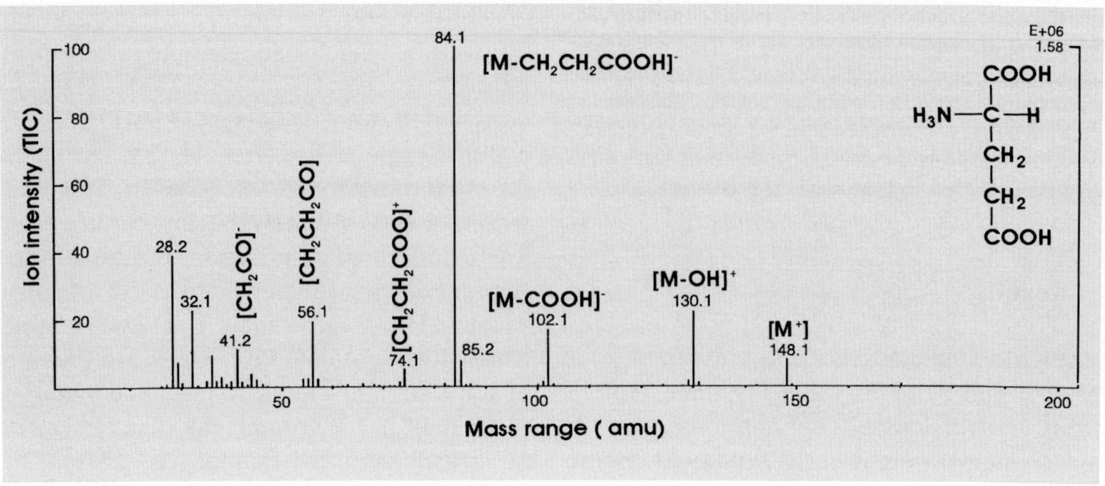

Fig. 5. EI-mass spectrum to confirm the fragment of *D-,L*-glutamic acid.

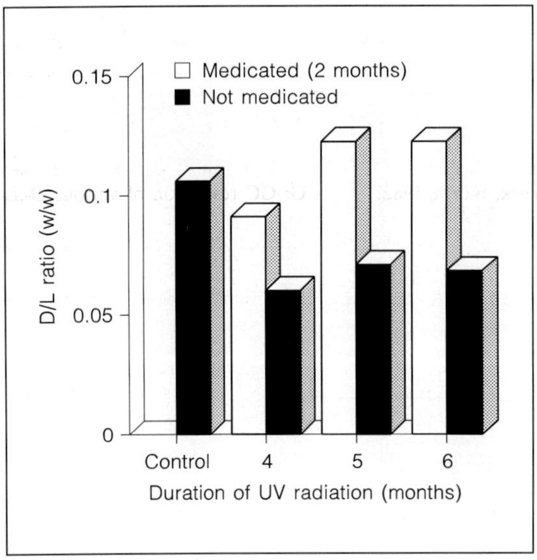

Fig. 6. Decrease of *D/L* ratio of glutamic acid in UV-B-induced cataract and the preventive effect of bendazac lysinate. (Analysis of control lenses was carried out after 6 months' duration.)

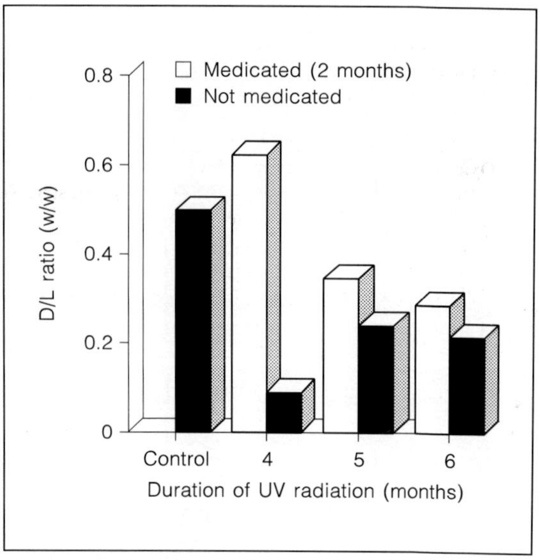

Fig. 7. Decrease of *D/L* ratio of lysine in UV-B-induced cataract and the preventive effect of bendazac lysinate. (Analysis of control lenses was carried out after 6 months' duration.)

rapid conversion of soluble to insoluble material. Therefore, the *D/L* ratio from the water-insoluble fraction of the cataractous lens is expected to be lower than in normal lens. Figure 6 shows the decrease in the *D/L* glutamic acid ratio by UV-B-induced cataract and the preventive effect of bendazac lysine.

The same decrease and the effect of medication were also observed in the case of lysine, as shown in figure 7. Provided that figures 6 and 7 are the results with no statistical test for significance due to the limitation of stereoisomers of amino acids from rat lens, these could be referred to as the methodology to evaluate or screen an effect of compounds.

Discussion

The *D/L* amino acid ratio from the water-insoluble fraction of UV-B-induced cataractous rat lenses is lower than that of normal rat lenses due to rapid transformation of water-soluble to -insoluble protein. This was shown for glutamic acid and lysine. The preventive action of bendazac lysine of this decrease was observed. The racemization of amino acids and changes in *D/L* ratio may contribute to the perturbation of protein structure, which may result in aggregation and insolubilization of lens protein, crystalline.

References

1 WHO: Management of Cataract in Primary Health Care Service. Geneva, World Health Organisation, 1990.

2 Young RW: Age-Related Cataract. Oxford, Oxford University Press, 1991.

3 He S, Pan S, Wu K, Amster IJ, Orlando R: Analysis of normal human fetal eye lens crystalline by HPLC/MS. J Mass Spect 1995;30:424–431.

4 Andley UP, Clarke BA: Generation of oxidants in the near UV photooxidation of human lens α-crystalline. Invest Ophthalmol Visual Sci 1989;30:706–713.

5 Hightower K, McCready J: Mechanisms involved in cataract development following near-ultraviolet radiation of cultured lens. Curr Eye Res 1992;11:679–689.

6 Lehninger AL: Principles of Biochemistry. New York, Worth, 1982.

7 Garner WH, Spector A: Racemization in human lens evidence of rapid insolubilization of specific polypeptide in cataract formation. Proc Natl Acad Sci USA 1978;75:3618–3620.

8 Pandolfo L, Livrea MA, Bono A: Effects of bendazac lysine salt on X-ray induced cataract in rabbit lens. Exp Eye Res 1986;42:167–175.

9 Cotlier E, Obara T, Toftness B: Cholesterol and phospholipids in protein fractions of human lens and senile cataract. Biochim Biophys Acta 1978;530:267–278.

10 Abe I, Izumi K, Kuramoto S, Muska G: GC resolution of various *D-,L-*amino acid derivatives on a chirasil-val capillary column. J HRC CC 1981;4:549–552.

11 Cheong JY, Choi SH, Woo NT, Shin JY, Kim SW, Jung WT: Racemization of l-lysine for pharmaceutical synthesis and its chiral separation by GC/MS spectroscopy. Arch Pharm Res 1995;18:69–74.

Ophthalmic Research

Ophthalmic Res 1996;28(suppl 2):32–36

K.P.Y. Foo
H. Maclean

Department of Ophthalmology,
Melbourne University,
Melbourne, Vic., Australia

Measured Changes in Cataract over Six Months: Sensitivity of the Nidek EAS-1000

Key Words
Cataract
Disease progression
Follow-up studies
Image analysis, computer-assisted
Lens cortex, crystalline
Lens nucleus, crystalline
Reproducibility of results
Scheimpflug photography
Retroillumination photography

Abstract
Lens opacities in 98 eyes from 63 consecutive outpatients with cataract were recorded by both retroillumination and Scheimpflug slit methods by one operator. This was repeated at 26 ± 1 weeks. Image analysis used the EAS-1000 software. Cortical and posterior subcapsular (PSC) cataracts were measured in retroillumination images as density more than 14 cct units below background density. Linear densitometry of white scattered light along the optical axis was measured for slit images by both peak density and mean density ('area under the curve'). Retroillumination images showed no discernible change over 6 months (the regression coefficient being as for the intersession reliability). Half of the Scheimpflug slit images could not be analysed because overlying cortical changes masked the more posterior parts of the lens. The other 49 eyes showed a significant increase in nuclear white scatter after 6 months, with greater degrees of change occurring in those eyes with the greatest amount of nuclear cataract initially. This is reflected by the decreased intraclass correlation coefficient (R = 0.42). The area of lens showing greatest change was the anterior fetal nucleus. The Nidek EAS-1000 is able to detect changes over a 6-month period in nuclear density but not in cortical or PSC cataract. The rate of progression of nuclear white scatter increases as the lens opacity becomes more dense. The ability to detect change in cataract over 6 months has implications for epidemiological studies and for trials of anti-cataract drugs.

KARGER

E-Mail karger@karger.ch
Fax + 41 61 306 12 34
http://www.karger.ch

© 1996 S. Karger AG, Basel
0030–3747/96/0288–0032$10.00/0

Dr. K.P.Y. Foo
Melbourne University
Department of Ophthalmology
32 Gisborne Street
East Melbourne, Vic. 3002 (Australia)

Introduction

Studies of the natural history of cataract and its possible modification by drugs require accurate measurement of the amount and location of lens opacities. Photographic methods of documenting cataract have been devised and improved over more than two decades. Clinical and photographic grading schemes have developed in parallel. The increasing capabilities of microcomputers directed attention to the application of image analysis techniques on lens photographs [1–15]. The most recent instruments use Charge Coupled Device cameras and allow immediate storage and analysis of digitised images. We report our experience with such an instrument [16] (Nidek EAS-1000) for medium-term follow-up of cataract.

Patients and Methods

Initial studies had explored the inter- and intra-observer and inter-session reproducibility of this camera. Those patients still attending who had participated in the Melbourne Catalin® trial [18] were invited to attend. Additional patients seen in routine outpatient practice who had identifiable cataract were invited to participate. Diabetics and those with glaucoma were excluded. The study was approved by the Human Research and Ethics Committee of our parent hospital. Informed consent was obtained from all patients. The cataracts were classified by one of us (H.M.) into cortical, nuclear, and posterior subcapsular (PSC) types. Many patients had one eye pseudophakic. 98 eyes from 63 patients were then imaged. Pupils were dilated with one drop each of proxymetacaine, tropicamide 0.5%, and phenylephrine 10% [19]. All eyes were re-imaged 6 months (± 1 week) later. All images were taken by the same operator (K.P.Y.F.). Camera settings were standardised. Retroillumination images were recorded using flash settings 2 and 3. That which gave a background brightness of between 110 and 170 was stored. Scheimpflug images also used 150 watt-second power, a 9-mm high vertical slit and the temporal location of the illuminator. Analysis of the digitised images was made using version 2.01a of the EAS-1000 software and only after completing taking the 6-month images. Analysis was done in masked fashion with no knowledge of which images were being analysed except where re-analysis was necessary for some retroillumination pictures because of differing pupil diameters. Retroillumination images were analysed according to a protocol previously described [20]. If there was a difference between initial and 6-month pictures, the smaller of the two diameters was used for both pictures. Scheimpflug images were measured by linear densitometry along the default optical axis. The central nuclear dip was readily recognisable. Peak density anterior (anterior fetal nucleus) and posterior to this (posterior fetal nucleus) was measured. For mean density ('area under the curve') the region from the dip to 1 mm posterior or 1 mm anterior to the central dip was analysed [9]. Analysis of variance was also performed using the SAS statistical package. From this, the intraclass correlation coefficient (R) was calculated (Appendix).

Results

Cortical Cataract and PSC Cataract (fig. 1a)

All 98 image pairs were analysed. There was no detectable change over 6 months (R = 0.99), but the amount of variability ('noise') inherent in the measurement is sufficient to obscure any small underlying trend.

Nuclear Cataract (fig. 1b–d)

A maximum of 49 eyes could be analysed. Nuclear change in the others was obscured by overlying cortical change and consecutive images did not give exactly the same optical section. The anterior fetal nucleus showed the greatest amount of change of peak density (R = 0.42) (fig. 1b). The posterior fetal nucleus change was similar with R = 0.46 from 47 eyes. The greater the initial density, with the exception of three nuclei that were found to be very deeply pigmented at operation, the greater the increase in density 6 months later (fig. 1c). The change in mean density of the anterior fetal nucleus is similar to that for peak density (R = 0.41) (fig. 1d).

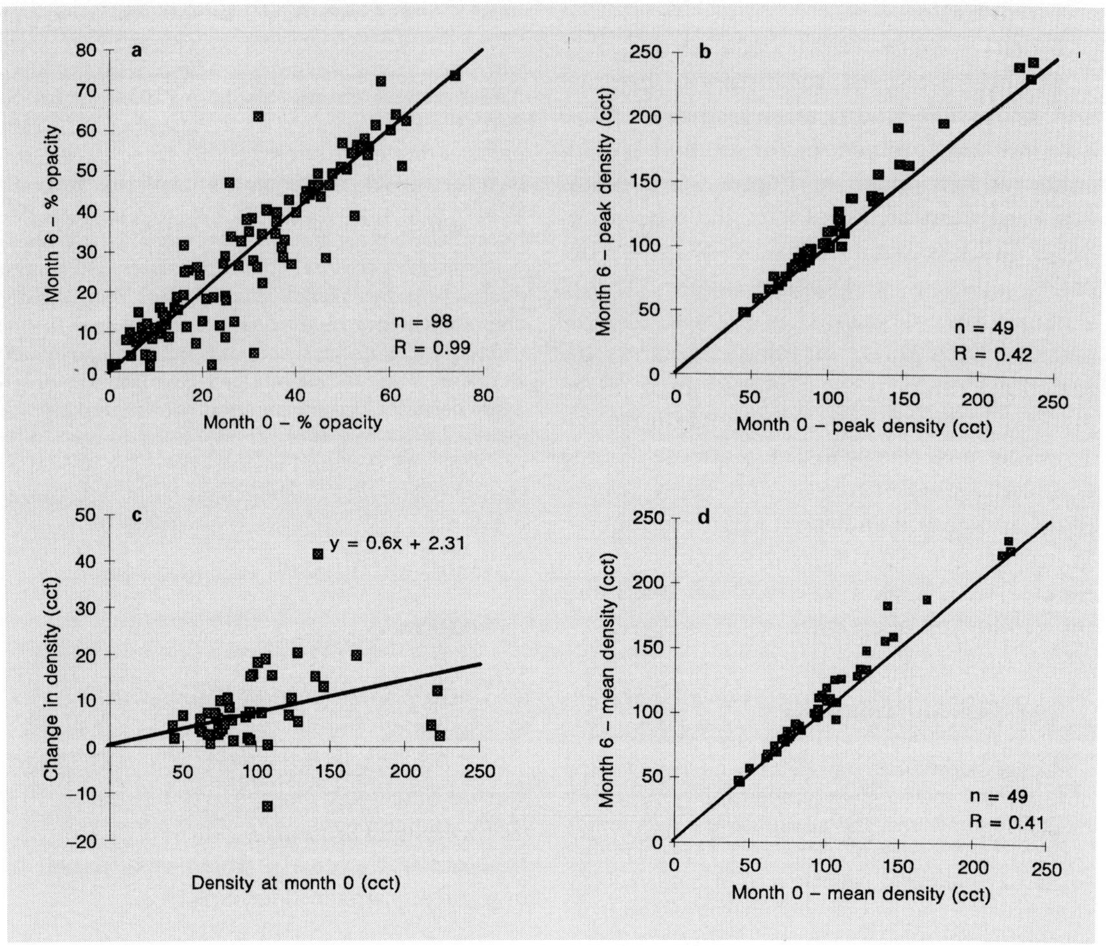

Fig. 1. a Analysis of retroillumination images for cortical and posterior subcapsular cataract at 0 and 6 months. There is no significant difference from the line of no change. The intraclass correlation coefficient (R) is the same as was found in earlier intersession reliability studies. **b** Peak density analysis for anterior fetal nucleus. The three outliers at the top right of the plot were found subsequently (when they came to surgery) to be particularly dark nuclei (cataracta nigricans). **c** Change in peak density of anterior fetal nucleus over 6 months. There is a greater increase in density in those nuclei where the initial density is higher. **d** Mean density of the anterior fetal nucleus. The plot is similar to that for peak density. Again the three dark nuclei appear as outliers.

Discussion

In the retroillumination picture comparisons, the intraclass correlation coefficient, R, indicates that there is no detectable change. It is the same value as found for intersession analyses in our reliability studies. Some of the 'noise' may be a reflection of small localised areas of improvement or worsening of cataract. A little may be due to the 'Maltese cross' effect from the cross polarisers in the camera interacting with the corneal birefringence [21,

22]. It is worth pointing out that the cortical change compares to that found with the original method of digital analysis from photographic transparency intermediates which suggested a 1-year increase of 1.6 ± 3.3% [7].

Cortical change can lead to nuclear obscuration in a number of ways. It may scatter too much light away from the nucleus leaving its illumination in the non-linear part of the CCD tube sensitivity curve. Very deeply pigmented nuclear cataracts may absorb so much back-scattered light and hence appear less dense. Additionally, even with the drops we used, some aged pupils dilated poorly and it was not possible to get good illumination of the posterior parts of the nucleus. High backscatter in the anterior fetal nucleus also decreases the amount of light transmitted to the more posterior parts of the nucleus and so makes them seem less dense than they really are. In practical terms, the anterior fetal nucleus is least affected by any of these changes and is the easiest to analyse.

Posterior subcapsular cataract has not been analysed separately but the small numbers have been included with the other retroillumination images of cortical opacities.

The use of 150 watt-seconds for the flash power settings was to prevent saturation of the CCD tube. Similarly, the height of the slit beam for Scheimpflug slit imaging was the maximum that could be used before the lashes, the eyebrows, and the structures of the chamber angle began to obtrude on the images and interfere with analysis.

The Nidek EAS-1000 camera is an instrument which will allow study of cataract progression and of its possible modification (medical intervention studies) within a realistic time frame. This applies particularly to the patients who have mainly nuclear cataracts.

Acknowledgments

Prof. H.R. Taylor for encouragement throughout, C. Carson and S. Lee for advice with statistical analysis, and RVEEH Research Committee for the optical storage system. During this work, K.P.Y. Foo was the recipient of the Hugh Noel Puckle scholarship from the University of Melbourne.

Appendix

Definition of intraclass correlation coefficient R:

$$R = \frac{\text{(between class mean square – within class mean square)}}{\text{(between class mean square + (k – 1)within class mean square)}},$$

where k = number of classes, in this case 2.

References

1 Chylack LT Jr, McCarthy D, Khu P: Use of Topcon SL-45 Scheimpflug slit photography to measure longitudinal growth of nuclear cataracts in vivo. Lens Res 1988;5:83–93.

2 Chylack LT Jr, McCarthy DF: How to avoid invalidation by changes in pupil size of longitudinal measures of cataract growth by retroillumination photography. Invest Ophthalmol Vis Sci 1987;28:323.

3 Harris ML, Hanna KJ, Shun Shin GA, Holden R, Brown NA: Analysis of retroillumination photographs for use in longitudinal studies of cataract. Eye 1993;7:572–577.

4 Harris ML, Smith GT, Brown NA: Inter- and intra-observer reproducibility of the new Oxford CCD Scheimpflug camera. Eye 1991;5: 487–490.

5 Hockwin O, Laser H, Kapper K: Image analysis of Scheimpflug negatives. Comparative quantitative assessment of the film blackening by area planimetry and height measurements of linear densitograms. Ophthalmic Res 1988;20:99–105.

6 Khu PM, Kashiwagi T: Quantitating nuclear opacification in color Scheimpflug photographs. Invest Ophthalmol Vis Sci 1993;34:130–136.

7 Maclean H, Taylor CJ: An objective staging for cortical cataract in vivo aided by pattern analysing computer. Exp Eye Res 1981:597–602.

8 Sasaki K, Fujisawa K, Sakamoto Y: Quantitative evaluation of nuclear cataract using image analysis. Ophthalmic Res 1992;24(suppl 1):26–31.

9 Sparrow JM, Brown NA, Shun Shin GA, Bron AJ: The Oxford modular cataract image analysis system. Eye 1990;4:638–648.

10 Van Den Broom HJB, Siertsema JV, Kooijman AC, Blanksma LJ, Van Rij G: Lens reflectometry with a CCD video camera and computer image analysis. Doc Ophthalmol 1991;78:237–244.

11 Datiles MB, Podgor MJ, Sperduto RD, Kashima K, Edwards P, Hiller R: Measurement error in assessing the size of posterior subcapsular cataracts from retroillumination photographs. Invest Ophthalmol Vis Sci 1989;30:1848–1854.

12 Hockwin O, Lerman S, Dragomirescu V: Image analysis of Scheimpflug photos of the lens by multiple linear microdensitometry. Lens Res 1984; 2:337.

13 Hockwin O, Dragomirescu V, Laser H: Measurements of lens transparency or its disturbances by densitometric image analysis of Scheimpflug photographs. Graefes Arch Clin Ophthalmol 1982;219:255–262.

14 Hockwin O, Dragomirescu V: Scheimpflug photography of the anterior eye segment: A method for measurement of lens transparency in long term studies. Excerpta Med Symp on the Lens, 1980, pp 62–76.

15 Sigelman J, Trokel SL, Spector A: Quantitative biomicroscopy of lens light back scatter: Changes in aging and opacification. Arch Ophthalmol 1974;92:437–442.

16 Sasaki K, Sakamoto Y, Shibata T: Application of an anterior eye segment analysis system in clinical cataract research. Lens Eye Tox Res 1990;7:505–515.

17 Foo KPY, Rule J, Golembo G, Lee SE, Maclean H, Taylor HR: Intraoperator, interoperator and intersession variability of the Nidek EAS-1000 for cataract quantification (abstract). Invest Ophthalmol Vis Sci. 1993;34:1223.

18 Maclean H: The Melbourne Catalin trial current protocol and some early results. Aust NZ J Ophthalmol 1977:183–187.

19 Maclean H: Reproducibility of mydriasis. Ophthalmic Res 1992;24 (suppl 1):36–39.

20 Foo KPY, Lee SE, Maclean H, et al: Quantification of cataract using the retroillumination module of the Nidek EAS-1000 anterior segment analysis system. Ophthalmic Res 1994;26(suppl 1):10–17.

21 Sakamoto Y, Rankov G, Sasaki K: Comparison of retroillumination images of crystalline lenses taken with different camera types. Ophthalmic Res 1990;22(suppl 1):41–45.

22 Kawara T, Obazawa H: A new method for retroillumination photography of cataractous lens opacities. Am J Ophthalmol 1980:186–189.

Ophthalmic Research

Ophthalmic Res 1996;28(suppl 2):37–44

D. Schweitzer
M. Hammer
M. Scibor

Department of Ophthalmology,
University of Jena, Germany

Imaging Spectrometry in Ophthalmology – Principle and Applications in Microcirculation and in Investigation of Pigments

Key Words
Imaging spectrometry
Fundus
Oxygen saturation
Melanin
Xanthophyll
Spectra deconvolution

Abstract
Imaging spectrometry is a new technique that permits simultaneous measurements of reflectance spectra at different locations along a line. Results are three-dimensional images, whose coordinates are location, wavelength, and reflectance. A conventional fundus camera is adapted to a spectrograph and an intensified charge coupled device (CCD) matrix detector system. The spectral resolution of this spectrometer is lower than 2 nm within a spectral range between 395 and 710 nm. The local resolution is lower than 23 µm along a line of 1.5 mm. From an imaging spectrum, the extinction spectrum of blood in vessels can be calculated. Also, in case of a noisy extinction spectrum of blood, its approximation by a model function results in calibration-free measurement of the oxygen saturation. Considering the radiation transport in single fundus layers, the local distribution of the concentration-thickness product of xanthophyll, melanin, and choroidal blood can be calculated.

Introduction

The value of spectrometric measurements of the eye was first demonstrated by the bleaching measurements of the photosensible receptor pigments [1, 2]. The fundus of the eye is illuminated by monochromatic light with a wavelength near the absorbance maximum of rhodopsin at 505 nm. The measurable double density of rhodopsin is the logarithm of the ratio of reflectances of the bleached and the dark adapted eye at a single wavelength.

KARGER

E-Mail karger@karger.ch
Fax + 41 61 306 12 34
http://www.karger.ch

© 1996 S. Karger AG, Basel
0030–3747/96/0288–0037$10.00/0

Doz. Dr. D. Schweitzer
Department of Ophthalmology
University of Jena
Bachstrasse 18
D–07740 Jena (Germany)

Whereas the first measurements were performed at single points, scanning laser ophthalmoscopy allows such measurements in the whole fundus plane [3, 4]. The double density of nonphotosensible pigments can also be calculated. In this case, reflectance is measured at a wavelength near the absorption maximum and at a wavelength at which the considered substance has no absorption. The local distribution of the macular pigment xanthophyll was measured in this way [5]. The extinction spectrum of a pigment can be measured if there is at least one location where this chromophore does not exist. If this is the case, the ratio of the reference location reflectance and of the measuring point is calculated for each wavelength within the measured spectrum [6]. The logarithm of this ratio is equivalent to the extinction spectrum of the considered pigment. In this calculation, besides the investigated pigment, comparable spectral properties are assumed at both locations. Caused by the eye movement, the comparison between reflectance spectra from different locations of the eye is very difficult.

If a complete reflectance spectrum is measured at a distinguished location, the optical double density of pigments in the sequence of fundus layers and the reflecting and scattering properties of interlayers can be calculated by spectra deconvolution [7–9].

Clinically relevant in the early diagnosis of glaucoma is the pallor of the optic disc, which is caused by a reduced erythrocyte content in the capillarized tissue [10, 11]. Glaucomatous alterations in the nerve fiber layer and in the microcirculation are detectable outside the optic disc as well [12, 13].

A further application of spectrometric investigations in the eye is the measurement for native fluorescence of the lens in cataract research [14] or in early detection of diabetes [15]. Fluorescence measurements of the orange-red component of lipofuscin are an essential tool to investigate the pathomechanism in age-related macular degeneration [16, 17].

Modern measuring techniques allow parallel measurement of the complete reflectance spectrum, simultaneously for a row of locations along a line. In this article the design of an imaging spectrometer and some applications for measurements of parameters characterizing dynamic or static aspects of the metabolism at the fundus are presented.

Table 1. Technical parameters of the imaging ophthalmospectrometer

Wavelength range, nm	395–710
Spectral resolution, nm	<2
Field size at the fundus, μm^2	1,500·40
Local resolution, μm	23
Optical density range	0–3.5
Optical density resolution at OD = 2	0.014
Standard deviation of flash, %	4
Exposure, μJ	36

OD = Optical density.

Method

Arrangement of an Imaging Ophthalmospectrometer

The imaging ophthalmospectrometer is based on a modified fundus camera (RCM 250, Carl Zeiss, Jena, Germany). A spectrograph (CP 200, Jobin-Yvon, Longjumeau, France) and an intensified CCD matrix camera (576S/RB, Princeton Instruments, Trenton, NY., USA) are adapted to the ophthalmoscope instead of the camera. The fundus is illuminated by a conventional xenon flash lamp. A slit-like field stop can be switched into the illuminating beam. The illuminated field at the fundus is 1.5 mm·40 μm. This field is confocally imaged onto the entrance slit of the spectrograph. The influence of the intraocular scattered light is reduced by the confocal imaging principle. The light, which originates from the fundus, is spectrally dispersed within the spectrograph. The intensified CCD

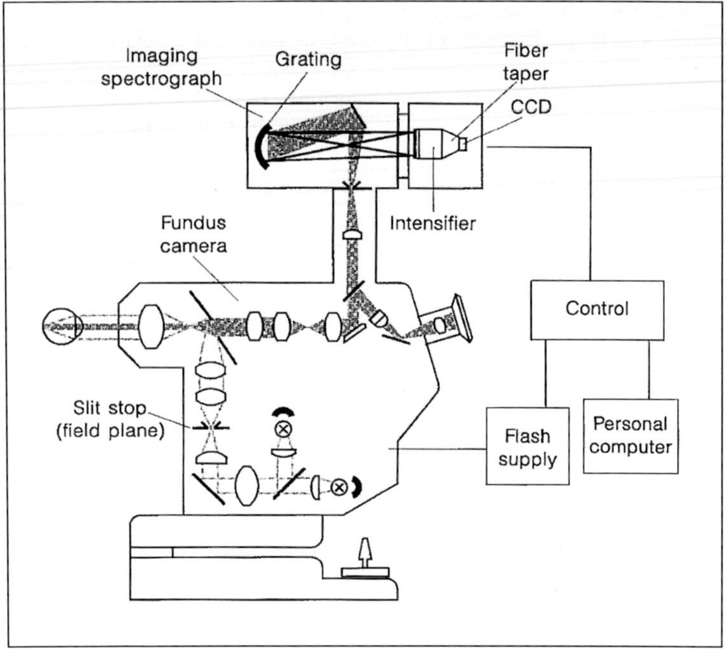

Fig. 1. Scheme of the imaging ophthalmospectrometer.

matrix camera detects a complete reflectance spectrum at the exit plane of the spectrograph in each line. In a column, the reflectance of the considered different locations at the same wavelength are presented. The imaging spectrum recorded is stored as two-dimensional image in a personal computer. The technical design of the computer-controlled spectrometer is drawn in figure 1. Table 1 shows the technical parameters of the spectrometer.

The advantage of this measuring principle is that the spectral information at all considered locations is measured at the same time. As the lens of the eye is located in the aperture plane, all beams of the measuring light, originating from different locations at the fundus, penetrate the lens in the same region. Thus the spectral transmission of the lens acts as a factor in all spectra at all locations. In the same way, fluctuations of the light intensity or different illumination conditions as a result of the eye movement also act as a constant factor for all wavelengths. Such influences are eliminated by normalization. Consequently, differences in the extinction between the considered locations can be measured very exactly, both independent of the measuring conditions at different times and independent of spectral characteristics of the light source or detector system. Because the ratio of the measured spectra is evaluated, the spectral characteristics of the light source, the detector system, and the spectral transmission of the optical system are without any influence.

In contrast, the calculation of the optical density of pigments in the sequence of single fundus layers by means of spectra deconvolution requires reflectance spectra. Reflectance spectra for each considered location are calculated after normalization to the imaging spectrum, which is detected from an artificial eye containing an ideal white Lambertian reflector (Spectralon, Labsphere Inc., reflectance 99%) in its focal plane. A solid angle correction between measurements of the human eye and of the artificial eye is necessary.

Examples for the Application of Imaging Spectrometry

Measurement of Microcirculation Parameters. Imaging spectrometry can be usefully applied for the investigation of retinal microcirculation. As spectral and local properties are measured in one step, the oxygen saturation and the diameter of vessels can be calculated on the basis of the imaging spectrum. The calibration-free measurement of oxygen saturation using imaging spectra was described by Schweitzer et al. [18]. The principle of this method is to calculate the extinction spectrum of blood in a first step as the logarithm of the ratio of the surrounding reflectance to the vessel reflectance. In a second step, such a calculated noise extinction spectrum of blood is approximated by a model function in a least-square algorithm. Besides the local distribution of the oxygen saturation, further data are calculated, which correspond to the concentration-thickness product of hemoglobin and of oxyhemoglobin.

In such measurements a low oxygen saturation between 30 and 40% was measured in retinal veins. The oxygen saturation in the arteries was always found to be higher than 80%. In small arteries, the calculated oxygen saturation was close to 100%.

This method was tested in an animal model as described by Schweitzer et al. [18]. In comparison with the results of a hemoxymeter (OSM 2, Radiometer, Copenhagen, Denmark) the oxygen saturation in small arteries and in venules of a neonatal porcine brain was within an error margin of ± 3%. Low oxygen saturation in human retinal veins was also measured by Delori [19].

In a second example oxygen saturation was measured in a cross-section through the fovea. The concentration-thickness product of hemoglobin is lower in the fovea than in its surroundings. This behavior corresponds to a decreased capillarization in the neighborhood of the fovea. In the capillary-free fovea, the residual values of the concentration-thickness product of both components of blood might belong to the choriocapillaris. In this measurement, the width of the capillary-free fovea is approximately 460 μm. The oxygen saturation in the neighborhood of the fovea is between 40 and 60%. In the capillary-free region it increases rapidly to values higher than 90%. It is assumed that this high oxygen saturation originates from the choriocapillaris, which supplies the receptors in the fovea.

The pallor of the optic disc is a mark of damaged microcirculation in glaucoma. The main parameters determining the pallor of the optic disc are the erythrocyte content in the capillarized tissue and the relation between reduced and oxidized hemoglobin. Both oxygen saturation and the erythrocyte content in the optic disc can be determined locally resolved using imaging spectrometry.

Measurements of Substance Spectra. For the identification of substances that exist as pathological alterations at the fundus, the extinction spectrum is a useful tool. An imaging spectrum of this local alteration and its surroundings contains all necessary information for this task. The logarithm of the ratio of the reflectance spectrum of the neighborhood to the reflectance spectrum at the local alteration results in the difference extinction spectrum. All components, equal in concentration at both locations, are eliminated. Therefore in some cases a reduced model function can be used for deconvolution of logarithmic difference spectra [13]. In this way it can be shown that the extinction spectrum of a nevus consists of both an increased extinction of melanin and a decreased extinction of blood in comparison with its neighborhood. A promising application is the deconvolution of logarithmic difference spectra, which are calculated between the reflectance at the papillomacular bundle and the fovea. This calculation results in information about differences in the locally distributed extinction of xanthophyll, melanin, and blood. As the sensitivity of the imaging spectrometer is very high, even local differences in the optical density of the ocular media are measurable in cataract cases.

It can be shown by imaging spectrometry that the contrast for the detection of bright hard exudates is optimal, if the fundus is illuminated by about 560 nm. As shown by Leistritz and Schweitzer [20], exact detection of the changed area of the exudates before and after coagulation is possible using the suitable wavelength in a scanning laser ophthalmoscope. The local distribution and the relative area of exudates are used both in diagnosis of diabetic retinopathy and for control of the effect of laser coagulation [20, 21].

Pigment Density in Different Fundus Layers. Figure 2 shows an imaging spectrum where the fovea is centred in the middle of the illuminated field. In this three-dimensional image one coordinate corresponds to the location of the measured points. The second axis is the wavelength between 395 and 710 nm. The vertical coordinate stands for the logarithm of the reflectance, which was measured at each location and at each wavelength. The reflectance at each location increases with higher wavelengths. The spectral course of the reflectance is predominantly the result of the absorption by melanin, by blood, and in the macular region by xanthophyll. In this imaging spectrum the central cup in the reflectance is caused by the absorption of xanthophyll.

Different models describe radiation transport in the layered fundus structures [7, 8, 22]. The basic idea of these models is that the initial radiation is more or less influenced by absorption, scattering and reflection in each single fundus layer. Thus the measurable light consists of a summation of different radiation fluxes, which originate from different layers. Using the known spectral courses of the absorption of pigments (e.g. melanin, xanthophyll, hemoglobin, oxyhemoglobin or receptor pigments) as well as the reflectance of the sclera or of scattering properties, the course of the measured spectrally dispersed light can be approximated

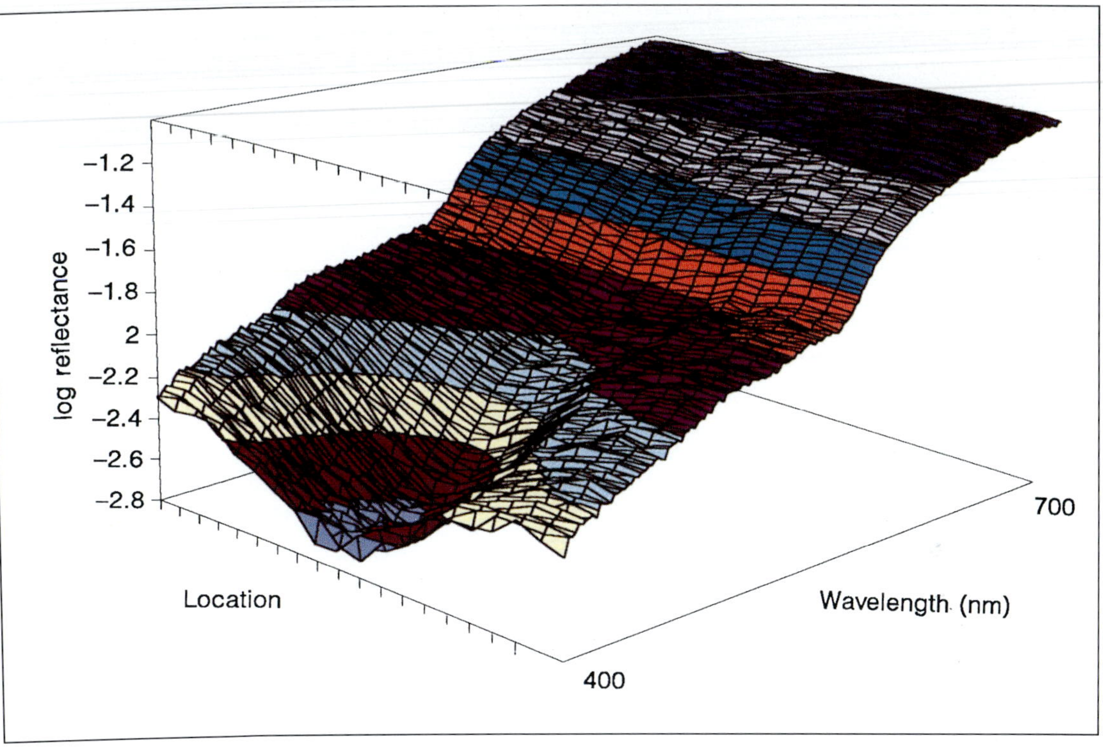

Fig. 2. Imaging spectrum of a cross-section through the fovea.

by a model function. In this least-square algorithm, parameters such as the concentration-thickness product of different chromophores, scattering properties and the reflection at intermediate layers and at the sclera are calculated.

A simple but sufficient model for the interaction of the illuminating light with the fundus was described by van Norren and Tiemeijer [7]. In this model, the reflected light consists of two radiation fluxes. The first part of the incident light which is reflected at the pigment epithelium is attenuated by the absorption of the ocular media and of the macular pigment xanthophyll. The second part of the light additionally penetrates the pigment epithelium and the choroid and is reflected at the sclera. During the double transmission, the reflected light is additionally diminished by the absorption of melanin and blood.

The spectrally reflected light in the macula can be approximated by the corresponding model function. Independent variables in the model function are the spectral extinction coefficients of the considered pigments, the spectral transmission of the ocular media, and the spectral reflectance of the sclera. In a least-square algorithm, the independent variables are weighted until the best fit is reached. The most important weight factors are the concentration-thickness products of the chromophores. As in imaging spectrometry, neighboring locations are investigated; therefore some influences can be assumed as similar in the model function of each considered point and a connected spectra deconvolution can be performed. As shown in figure 3, the local distribution of pigments, for example xanthophyll, melanin, or choroidal blood, can be calculated. Such quantitative information about the layered fundus structures can lead to an improved diagnosis, for example in diabetic retinopathy and in evaluating the effect of laser therapy.

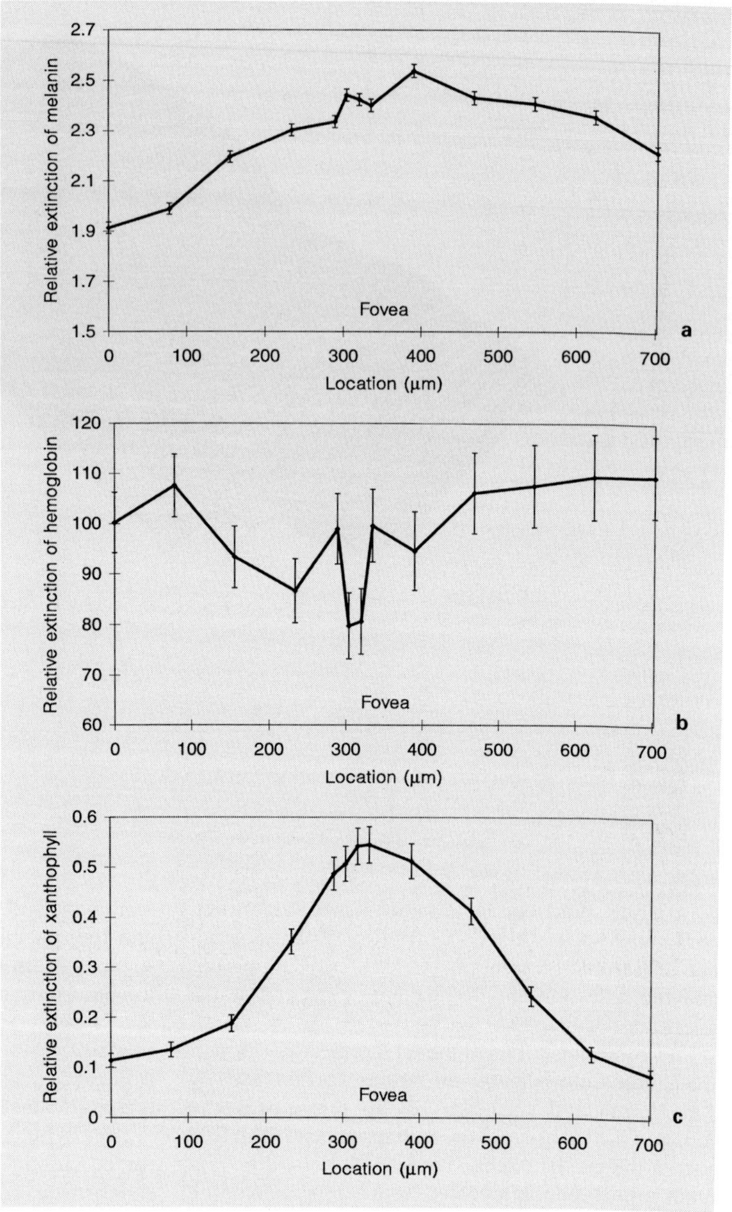

Fig. 3. Local distribution of single chromophores, measured in a healthy macula. **a** Absorbance of melanin, normalized to the absorbance of retinal pigment epithelium as measured by Gabel et al. [23]. **b** Thickness in micrometers of an equivalent layer of hemoglobin solution (concentration 150 g/l). **c** Absorbance of xanthophyll, normalized to the values given by Wyszecki and Stiles [24].

Discussion

Spectrometric measurements are limited by the maximal permissible exposure of the fundus [25]. Using the illumination system of commercial fundus cameras, the signal-noise ratio is only in the order of 50, indicating high uncertainty of measurements at single wavelengths. If a large number of wavelengths is evaluated in parallel, the signal-noise ratio requirements are reduced in the order of the square root of the considered wavelengths. The advantage of imaging spectrometry consists in the simultaneous measurement of the reflectance spectra of neighboring locations. In this way, the influence of eye movements in calculation of local spectral differences is reduced. A rather promising application of imaging spectrometry is the simultaneous measurement both of oxygen saturation in arteries as well as veins and of vessel diameter. These parameters are important to describe alterations in microcirculation. From first results, it can be concluded that the consumption of oxygen in the retina is very high. About 50% of oxygen in the arteries is utilized in the tissue. The oxygen saturation in retinal veins (approximately 40%) is much lower than the oxygen saturation in other veins. This principal relation is common knowledge as is the Pasteur effect; the mutual inhibition of respiration and glycolysis does not exist in the retina [26]. The measured different gradients of oxygen saturation in the tissue between arteries and veins remain to be interpreted in the future.

The measurement of the reflectance spectra of locally distributed pigments allows the determination of the optimal illumination wavelength for the highest contrast in visualization or measurement by laser scanning ophthalmoscopy.

The connected spectra deconvolution permits the quantitative calculation of absorbing or scattering structures in the layered fundus. Such calculations might be important in the evaluation of the extension and the density of an edema, for example in diabetic retinopathy. In this case, the scattering of light within an edema should be changed in comparison with its surroundings.

In the early stage of age-related macular degeneration, a growing membrane under the pigment epithelium is assumed. This change should also be measurable by imaging spectrometry. Further applications of imaging spectrometry are the detection and differentiation of nevi and tumors, if they have different spectral properties.

Using a lens in front of the ophthalmoscope, corresponding to the optical properties of the human eye, the imaging spectrometer can also be used for the investigation of the anterior part of the eye. Whereas the spectral properties of the iris are easily measurable by the described arrangement, the locally resolved fluorescence or scattering of the lens should be performed using a slit lamp as the basic device.

References

1. Weale RA: Photochemical reactions in the living cat's retina. J Physiol 1953;12:322–331.
2. Rushton WAH: The difference spectrum and the photosensitivity of rhodopsin in the living human eye. J Physiol 1956;134:11–29.
3. van Norren D, van der Kraats J: Imaging retinal densitometry with a confocal scanning laser ophthalmoscope. Vision Res 1989;29:1825–1830.
4. Elsner AE, Burns SA, Huges GW, Webb RH: Reflectometry with the scanning laser ophthalmoscope. Appl Opt 1992;31:3697–3710.
5. Kilbride PE, Alexander K, Fishman M, Fishman GA: Human macular pigment assessed by imaging fundus reflectometry. Vision Res 1989;29:663–674.
6. Schweitzer D, Klein S, Stein A, Truckenbrodt C: Glaukomdiagnostik mittels Fundusspektrometrie in Bereichen ausserhalb der Papille. Klin Monatsbl Augenheilkd 1991, 198:544–549.
7. van Norren D, Tiemeijer LF: Spectral reflectance of the human eye. Vision Res 1986;26:313–320.
8. Delori FC, Pflibsen KP: Spectral reflectance of the human ocular fundus. Appl Opt 1989;28:1061–1077.

9 Schweitzer D, Königsdörffer E, Tröger G, Augsten R, Klein S, Roth H: Möglichkeiten und Grenzen der Fundusreflektometrie zum Nachweis von Veränderungen in einzelnen Schichten des Augenhintergrundes. Folia Ophthalmol 1990;15: 125–137.
10 Zenker HJ, Mierdel P, Marré E: Quantitative evaluation of pallor-disc ratio and color of the optic disc by photographic method. Graefes Arch Clin Exp Ophthalmol 1983; 220:184–186.
11 Schwartz B, Takamoto T, Nagin P: Measurement of reversibility of optic disc cupping and pallor in ocular hypertension and glaucoma. Ophthalmology 1985;92:1396–1407.
12 Knighton RW, Jacobson SG, Kemp CM: The spectral reflectance of the nerve fiber layer of the macaque retina. Invest Ophthalmol Vis Sci 1989;30:2393–2402.
13 Schweitzer D, Günther S, Scibor M, Hammer M: Spectrometric investigations in ocular hypertension and early stages of primary open angle glaucoma and of low tension glaucoma – Multisubstance analysis. Int Ophthalmol 1992;16:251–257.
14 Hemenger RP, Occhipinti JR: Aging parameters of the ocular lens by scanning fluorophotometry. Ophthalmic Physiol Opt 1989;9:191–197.
15 Larsen M, Kjer B, Bendtson I, Dalgaard P, Lund-Andersen H: Lens fluorescence in relation to nephropathy in insulin-dependent diabetes mellitus. Graefes Arch Clin Exp Ophthalmol 1992;230:6–10.
16 Delori FC, Dorey KC, Staurenghi G, Arend O, Goger DC, Weiter JJ: In vivo fluorescence of the ocular fundus exhibits retinal pigment epithelium lipofuscin characteristics. Invest Ophthalmol 1995;36:718–729.
17 von Rückmann A, Fitzke FW, Bird AC: Distribution of fundus autofluorescence with a scanning laser opthalmoscope. Br J Ophthalmol 1995;79:407–412.
18 Schweitzer D, Leistritz L, Hammer M, Scibor M, Bartsch U, Strobel J: Calibration-free measurement of the oxygen saturation in retinal vessels of men; in Parel J-M, Ren Q, Joos KM (eds): Ophthalmic Technologies. V. Progress in Biomedical Optic. SPIE Proc Ser. Bellingham, SPIE, 1995, vol 2393, pp 210–218.
19 Delori FC: Noninvasive technique for oxymetry of blood in retinal vessels. Appl Opt 1989;27:1113–1125.
20 Leistritz L, Schweitzer D: Automated detection and quantification of exudates in retinal images; in Tescher AG (ed): Applications of Digital Image Processing. SPIE Proc Ser. Bellingham, SPIE, 1994, vol 2298, pp 690–696.
21 Phillips R, Forrester J, Sharp P: Automated detection and quantification of retinal exudates. Graefes Arch Clin Exp Ophthalmol 1993; 231:90–94.
22 Schweitzer D, Tröger G, Königsdörffer E, Klein S: Multisubstanzanalyse – Nachweis von Änderungen der optischen Dichte in einzelnen Schichten des Augenhintergrundes. Fortschr Ophthalmol 1991; 88:554–561.
23 Gabel VP, Birngruber R, Hillenkamp F: Visible and near infrared light absorption in pigment epithelium and choroid. XXIII Concilium Ophthalmologicum, Kyoto. Amsterdam, Excerpta Medica, 1978.
24 Wyszecki G, Stiles WS: Color Science. New York, Wiley, 1967.
25 American National Standard for the Safe Use of Laser ANSI Z 136.1-1980.
26 Krebs H: Der Pasteur-Effekt und die Beziehung zwischen Atmung und Gärung in lebenden Zellen. Naturwissenschaftl Rundsch 1972;25: 387–393.

Ophthalmic Research

Ophthalmic Res 1996;28(suppl 2):45–53

John L. Hess[a]
Kenneth P. Mitton[b]
G.E. Bunce[a]

[a] Department of Biochemistry and Anaerobic Microbiology, Virginia Polytechnic Institute and State University, Blacksburg, Va., and
[b] National Eye Institute, National Institutes of Health, Bethesda, Md., USA

Precataractous Changes Affect Lens Transparency in the Selenite Cataract

Key Words
Cataract model
Crystallin
Glutathione
Lens
Phase separation
Rat
Selenite

Abstract

Selenite treatment of the preweanling rat stabilized the transparency of the lens nucleus to decreasing temperature. Hence, we compared properties of the cortex and nucleus from lenses of selenite-treated and age-matched control rats. A subcutaneous dose of 30 nmol Na_2SeO_3/g body weight was administered to 10- to 13-day-old Sprague-Dawley rats. Uninjected, age-matched littermates served as controls. As required, lenses were frozen in liquid N_2 and separated into nuclear and cortical-epithelial fractions. Transparency of solutions of lens proteins (90–100 mg per ml) was monitored from 30 to 2 °C as percent transmittance (%T) at 490 nm. The critical phase separation temperature, T_c, was the temperature at 80%T. Protein associations were monitored with gel filtration chromatography. The nuclear 'cold cataract', in intact lenses, formed at similar temperatures at 14 and 15 days of age, but at a significantly lower temperature when the lenses were from a selenite-treated rat. The T_c, however, was greater by 1.5–2 °C for solutions of proteins isolated from whole lenses or lens nuclei from rats 24 and 48 h after treatment with selenite. Further, less γ-crystallin was associated with the α-crystallin fraction in extracts from the nucleus of lenses from treated rats. Altered phase separation properties occurred as an early event in the etiology of selenite cataract. The different in vivo and in vitro responses to temperature indicated that properties of lens crystallins do not solely establish transparency in the intact lens.

Introduction

Cataract may result from molecular damage caused by increased oxidative stress in the lens. In rats a systemic dose of Na_2SeO_3 results in nuclear cataract formation [1, 2]. Among the changes that precede nuclear cataract formation are the formation of a transient posterior subcapsular opacity (PSO) [3], decreased glutathione content in the lens [2, 4], and altered temperature-dependent phase transition properties of the lens [5, 6].

Nuclear opacification occurs reversibly in vitro as the temperature of the neonate rat

KARGER

E-Mail karger@karger.ch
Fax + 41 61 306 12 34
http://www.karger.ch

© 1996 S. Karger AG, Basel

John L. Hess
Department of Biochemistry and Anaerobic Microbiology
Virginia Polytechnic Institute and State University
Blacksburg, VA 24061-0308 (USA)

lens is decreased from 37 to 25 °C. For lenses from control rats this change begins around 32 °C, while for lenses from selenite-treated animals the nucleus remains transparent until the temperature reaches 28 °C. It has been established that this relative difference contradicted the phase separation properties of solutions containing proteins from these lenses [6]. Low-molecular-weight polyions such as amino acids can stabilize the phase separation properties of concentrated crystallin solutions [6, 7]. Hence, altered lens transparency results from the interaction of multiple factors that may vary in different regions of the lens.

We have completed these experiments to determine the extent to which localized changes in the lens contribute to the temperature sensitivity of transparency in lenses from control and selenite-treated rats. Specific comparisons are presented for properties of proteins between the nuclear and cortical regions of lenses.

Methods

Cataract Induction

Sprague-Dawley rats were housed in polypropylene shoebox cages and fed Agway 3000 laboratory rat chow (Agway Inc. C.G., Syracuse, N.Y., USA) and distilled water. Ten- to 13-day-old rats were injected subcutaneously with 20 m*M* Na_2SeO_3 0.9% NaCl for a total dose of 30 nmol g^{-1} body weight (approximately 30 µl injection). Control animals from the same litter, but not injected [2], were used for all experiments. All experiments adhered to the ARVO Statement for the Use of Animals in Ophthalmic and Vision Research.

Isolation of Lens Nuclear/Cortex Tissue

At designated times after injection, animals were decapitated and lenses were removed immediately for extraction of metabolites or proteins. Lens cortical and nuclear tissue were obtained by dissecting liquid N_2 frozen lenses [6]. Intact lenses, bathed in 0.9% NaCl, were observed and photographed at different temperatures with an Olympus SZH zoom-stereo microscope equipped with a model SZH-ILLD illumination base (Olympus Optical Co., Tokyo, Japan).

Total Soluble Protein Extract

Lenses, frozen using liquid N_2, were stored at −80 °C in order to obtain sufficient tissue (22 lenses/extract) for the protein extraction in 100 m*M* NaH_2PO_4, 5.0 m*M* EDTA, 0.01% NaN_3, adjusted to pH 7.20 (295 mosm) [6]. The homogenate was warmed to 15–17 °C during the homogenization. Samples from selenite-treated rats were processed simultaneously with their controls. Experiments were repeated three times.

Protein Determinations

Protein content was measured using the dye-binding assay of Bradford [8]. Bovine serum albumin was the standard.

Phase Separation Temperature Curves

Phase separation was monitored at 490 nm as percent transmittance (%T) of protein samples at various temperatures [6]. Samples were diluted with dialysis buffer to equivalent protein concentration (91 or 96 mg ml^{-1}). Light transmission was monitored from high to low temperature after equilibrating samples for 1.5 min at a new set temperature. All solutions were transparent at 36 °C and were referenced to 100%T at this temperature. Solution turbidity was stable and visually apparent at 80%T (490 nm), and used as the measure of the critical temperature (T_c, °C). Statistical comparisons, using the Duncan multiple-range test [9], were based on the average T_c calculated from this most stable region of transmittance change betwen 76 and 90%T. Once light transmission fell below 75%T, transmittance even at constant temperature decreased continuously.

Gel Filtration Chromatography

An analytical Bio-Sil SEC-250 column (BioRad, USA) was equilibrated at room temperature with a mobile phase of 0.1 *M* Na_2SO_4 and 0.02 *M* NaH_2PO_4 at pH 6.8. The flow rate of 1 ml min^{-1} provided separation of standards from 670 to 1.3 kD within 15 min. Absorbance was monitored at 210 nm. Samples of the soluble protein fraction, prepared from the nucleus and cortex/epithelium fraction, were loaded at 100 µg total protein. Protein concentrations of the sample solutions, maintained at room temperature in the extraction buffer, were adjusted from 2.5 to 20 mg protein ml^{-1}. Sample volumes on the column varied between 2.5 and 40 µl. These conditions were established with solutions of bovine serum albumin that revealed a constant distri-

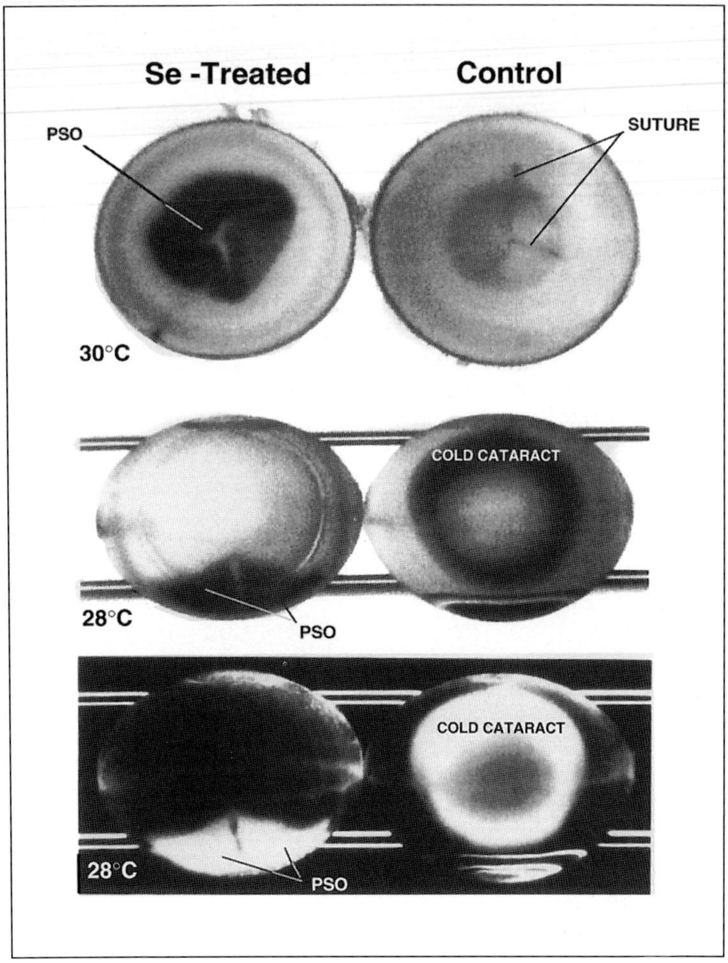

Fig. 1. Lenses from age-matched control and selenite-injected rats, 48 h after treatment. Top: posterior view of lenses from age-matched control (right) and treated (left) rats bathed in 0.9% NaCl at 30 °C under bright-field illumination. The control lens shows initial stages of 'cold cataract' formation in the lens nuclear region, while the treated lens displays only the PSO that is oriented about the posterior suture. Center: equatorial view of the same lenses supported on glass rods, separated by 1.75 mm, in saline at 28 °C under bright-field illumination. The control lens displays a nuclear 'cold cataract' now more obvious than at 30 °C. The corresponding nuclear region of the lens from treated animals is clear. The anterior surface is oriented upward so that the PSO now appears as the opacity in the lower area of the lens. The typical discontinuity in light refraction, seen as a ring about the perinuclear region, is visible in the lens from the treated group. Bottom: dark-field illumination of the same lenses shown in the center panel enhances the contrast of light-scattering areas (white) and transparent areas (black).

bution between the high- and low-molecular-weight aggregates characteristic of serum albumin.

Results

Appearance of the Lens

In figure 1 we present both a posterior and a side view of a typical lens from control and from selenite-treated rats 48 h after treatment with selenite, prior to nuclear cataract formation. A temperature-insensitive PSO forms within 24 h and disappears as the lens develops. It is no longer present at the time nuclear opacity occurs between 72 and 96 h after treating animals with selenite [3]. Above 30 °C the nuclear region of all lenses is transparent. However, at 28 °C age-matched control lenses have an obvious nuclear 'cold cataract', although none occurs at this temperature in lenses from selenite-treated rats 24–48 h after treatment. The temperature must be decreased to 24 °C in order for the lens from selenite-treated animals to form a 'cold cataract' similar to the opacity routinely observed in control animals at 28 °C.

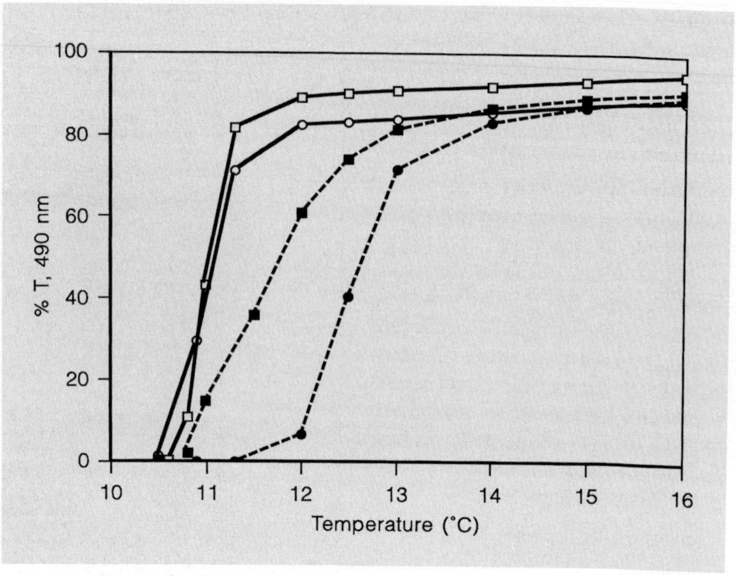

Fig. 2. Phase separation properties of total soluble lens proteins in vitro. Solutions, containing 96.8 mg protein ml^{-1} in 300-mosm buffer, were prepared from soluble proteins extracted from lenses of age-matched control and selenite-treated rats 24 and 48 h after treatment. Light transmission (%T) at 490 nm was plotted as a function of solution temperature, control responses (open symbols on solid lines) and treated responses (solid symbols on dashed lines). Circles are for data from lenses 24 h after treatment and squares are for the data from lenses 48 h after treatment.

Phase Separation Comparisons

In figures 2 and 3 we present temperature-dependent transparency measurements for extracts from the whole lens and from the nucleus and cortex of lenses from selenite-treated and age-matched control rats. The T_c for these solutions was higher for the samples derived from the lenses exposed to selenite. Further, protein solutions from the nucleus scattered more light at higher temperatures compared to the cortex (fig. 3). Estimations of T_c for all these samples are presented in table 1. These results are unexpected [5] since, as shown in figure 1, 'cold cataract' forms at a lower temperature in lenses from selenite-treated rats compared to age-matched, control rats. On the other hand, transparency was maintained at lower temperatures for protein solutions prepared from the cortex fraction of lenses from selenite-treated rats. This response is consistent with the properties of the intact lens.

Association of γ-Crystallin with α-Crystallin

Gel filtration chromatography of soluble proteins from the lens yielded three major regions on the chromatogram that accounted for 98% of the total peak area. We defined these areas as: α-crystallin (500–200 kD), β-crystallin (150–40 kD), and γ-crystallin (20 kD). Simple HPLC gel filtration experiments revealed a concentration-dependent association of γ-crystallin with proteins included in the α-crystallin fraction as shown in figure 4. As protein concentrations increased from 2.5 to 20 mg ml^{-1}, the increase in the proportion of α-crystallin corresponded to a decrease in the γ-crystallin fraction for extracts from the nucleus (fig. 4A) and from the cortex (fig. 4B). Hence, the content of γ-crystallin at 56% in the nucleus decreased to 48% as the protein concentration increased eightfold. For the cortex over this same concentration range the γ-crystallin decreased from 42 to 30%. The relative amount of intermediate-

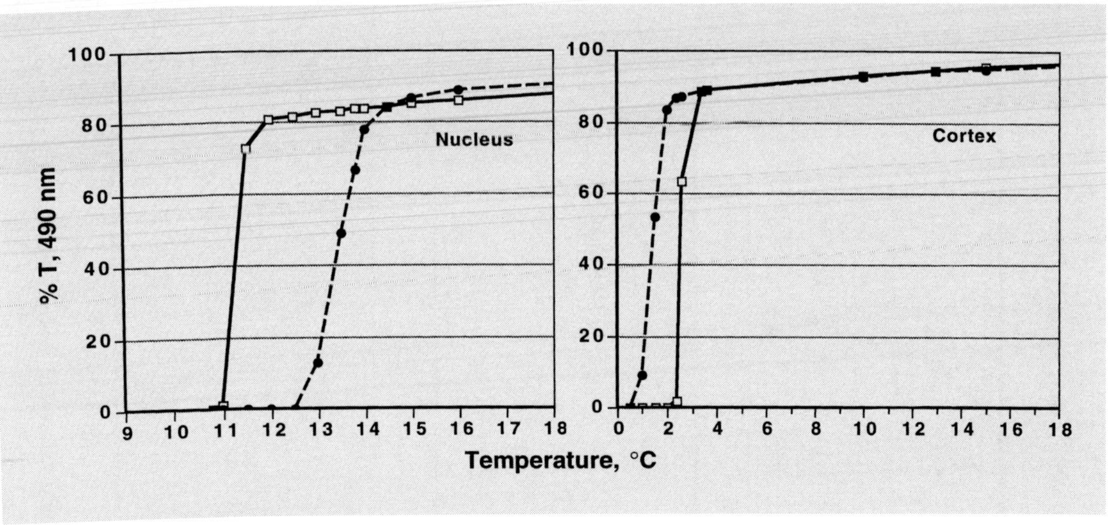

Fig. 3. Phase separation properties in vitro of soluble proteins isolated from lens cortex and nucleus. Light transmission at 490 nm (%T) was plotted as a function of solution temperature. Solutions, containing 91.0 ± 1 mg protein ml^{-1} in 300-mosm buffer, were prepared from soluble proteins extracted from the cortex and nucleus of lenses from age-matched control (solid line, open circle) and selenite-treated rats 48 h after treatment (dashed line, solid square).

Table 1. Apparent T_c of solutions of proteins isolated from lenses of selenite-treated rats compared to similar solutions from lenses of age-matched control rats

Time after treatment h	Animal age days	T_c, °C[1] at 80% T control	selenite-treated	average (76–90%T) control	selenite-treated
24	14	11.5	13.9	13.9	14.7
48	15	11.3	12.9	11.7	13.9
48	15				
Nucleus		11.7	14.0		
Cortex		2.4	1.8		

1 For solutions containing 96 ± 1 mg protein ml^{-1}, values of T_c at 80%T were estimated from the phase separation curves in figures 2 and 3. Experiments were repeated one time. The average T_c was calculated for 7 temperatures determining 76–90%T. The average T_c for solutions of protein from lenses of selenite-treated rats was significantly higher than for solutions of protein from lenses of control rats ($p < 0.05$). The average T_c for the samples from lenses of 14-day-old animals (24 h after treatment) was significantly higher compared to the comparable sample from 15-day-old rats (48 h after treatment, $p < 0.01$).

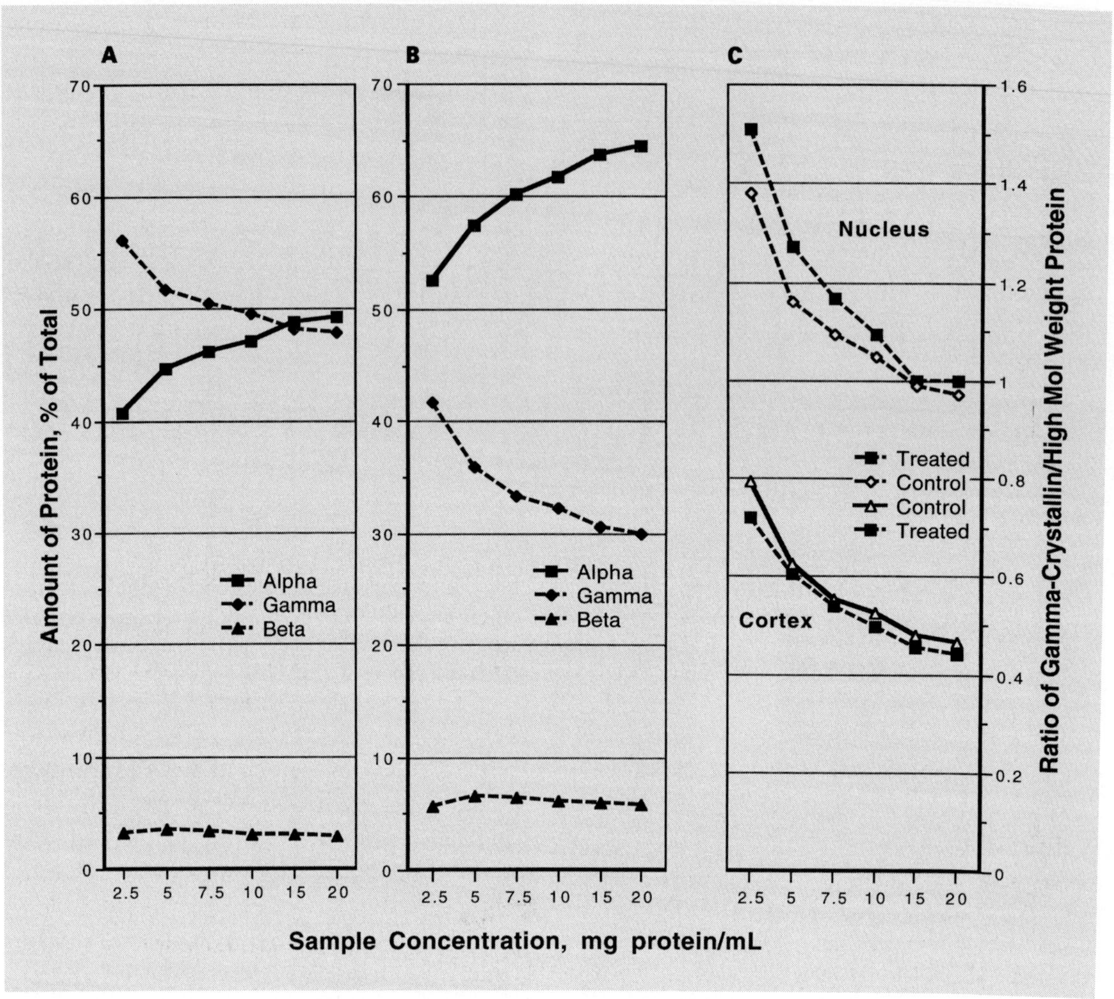

Fig. 4. Concentration-dependent distribution of soluble proteins among three major fractions obtained from HPLC chromatography of protein extracts from the nucleus or cortex of lenses. All samples were applied as 100 μg total protein and chromatographed under standard conditions on a Bio-Sil SEC-250 column with a flow rate of 1 ml min^{-1}. Absorbance of effluent was measured at 210 nm. Quantities of protein in three major peaks, α-crystallin, β-crystallins, and γ-crystallin, were compared. Samples contained from 2.5 to 20 mg protein ml^{-1}. Areas for each fraction, as a percent of the total area of the chromatogram, were plotted as a function of protein concentration in the sample. Total recovery for three experiments varied by 8 ± 2%. Distributions were plotted for proteins from the cortex (**A**) and nucleus (**B**) of lenses from control rats. **C** Data are plotted as the ratio of free γ-crystallin content to content of α-crystallin at each concentration for protein extracted from lenses of age-matched control and selenite-treated rats 48 h after treatment.

molecular-weight proteins, β-crystallins, was unaffected by the protein content of the sample.

Comparisons of this concentration-dependent property of γ-crystallin to associate with higher-molecular-weight aggregates are plotted in figure 4C and include data for extracts from lenses of selenite-treated and from age-matched control rats. For samples prepared from the nucleus of lenses from selenite-treated rats at less than 7 mg protein ml^{-1}, less γ-crystallin associated with the α-crystallin fraction. In extracts from the lens cortex, no significant difference was apparent in response to selenite treatment.

Discussion

Prior to the occurrence of nuclear cataract, formation of 'cold cataract' requires a lower temperature for intact lenses from selenite-treated rats compared to lenses from age-matched controls [5, 6]. This different response to temperature is readily observed as shown in figure 1. The initial increase in light scattering appears at the interface between the nucleus and the cortex. This change occurs only when the temperature is 4°C lower in lenses from selenite-treated rats compared to those from controls. At this early stage of 'cold cataract' the interior of the nucleus remains transparent, although 'cold cataract' involves the entire nucleus as the temperature decreases further.

As expected [4], total glutathione uniformly and significantly decreased in both the nucleus and the cortex of the lenses from selenite-treated rats at this early stage of pathology (data not shown). The selective effects that result in a nuclear 'cold cataract' and the differential temperature sensitivity between lenses from selenite-treated and those from age-matched control rats was not caused by specific regional perturbations in glutathione content.

Recall that 'cold cataract' forms at a lower temperature in lenses from selenite-treated rats compared to age-matched controls (fig. 1). It was therefore expected that the phase separation for concentrated protein solutions derived from lenses exposed to selenite would occur at a lower temperature as well. As reported in figures 2 and 3, phase separations in these solutions from the whole lens and the nucleus occur at a higher temperature in response to selenite treatment. As expected from measurements made with solutions of bovine crystallin [10], the γ-crystallin-rich nuclear fraction proteins had a higher T_c than observed for the cortical fraction (fig. 3, table 1).

As reported by Mitton et al. [6] significant increases occur in the free amino acid content of lenses from selenite-treated rats by 24 h after selenite treatment and that these changes occurred in both the nucleus and the cortex of the lens. Further, they observed that the addition of amino acids at concentrations equivalent to those in the lens caused the phase separation of solutions of protein from the rat lens to occur at a higher temperature. Hammer and Benedek [7] have also reported similar effects for solutions of protein from the calf lens.

Since all of the light-scattering measurements were performed on dialyzed solutions, differences in the T_c for these solutions must reflect differences in protein composition or differences caused by modification of proteins. The gel-filtration-chromatographic separations at different protein concentrations were used to explore how the capacity for proteins to assemble into larger-molecular-weight aggregates may be affected by the exposure of lenses to selenite. Solutions of bovine serum albumin, over this concentration range and amount of protein, had a constant ratio of

Hours (after treatment)	METABOLIC CHANGES	PHYSICAL CHANGES	Cataract
0	ATP levels lower		
12	Pentose pathway flux increase	DNA damage	
	Free amino acids increase		
24	Glutathione (40% of control)		PSO
		Altered phase separation properties	
36	NADP$^+$/NADPH increase	**Altered Crystallins (?)**	
	Glycerol phosphate maximum	Discontinuity in cortex diffraction	
48		Extracellular space increase	
	Elevated calcium content		
72	Metabolism recovering	Calpain dependent proteolysis of crystallins	
96			Nuclear

Fig. 5. Summary of some events that precede nuclear opacity in the selenite-treated cataract model. The times after treating preweanling rats with selenite appear on the left. The general appearance of the lens at 24 and 96 h is noted on the right. Comparisons are summarized from earlier work in our laboratory and others [2, 3, 4, 6, 13, 14].

high-low-molecular-weight associations (data not shown). For the proteins from lenses, the distribution was essentially biphasic with a high-molecular-weight α-crystallin fraction and a low-molecular-weight γ-crystallin fraction. No age-dependent very high-molecular-weight (>600 kD) fraction occurred in these very young rodent lenses in agreement with the data of Russell et al. [11] for the mouse (BALBc).

As the protein concentration was increased in samples prepared from the cortex, more γ-crystallin associated with the α-crystallin fraction compared to that occurring in extracts from the nucleus. This difference reflected the greater amount of α-crystallin in the cortex available for binding. These interactions were detected only at protein concentrations greater than 2 mg ml^{-1} and revealed different protein-protein associations and how modifications to proteins will impact the stability of α-/γ-crystallin assemblies.

These results establish that early changes in the soluble protein populations must occur. However, by themselves these changes do not explain the nuclear transparency at lower temperature that characterize the intact lens from selenite-treated rats prior to nuclear cataract formation. It is the organization of these proteins in the presence of millimolar concentrations of metabolites that contributes to the overall response to temperature. Hiraoka and Clark [12] prevented nuclear cataract formation in the selenite model using phase separation inhibitors such as pantethine. How such agents may affect the precataractous phase separation properties of the soluble proteins is not known.

We do not consider that these modifications are necessarily related to accelerated proteolysis [13]. Calcium content becomes significantly elevated only 48 h after selenite treatment [14] and may not be a factor in these early precataractous changes.

The role of α-crystallin as a molecular chaperone has been demonstrated. These crystallins can protect proteins against denaturation caused by increased temperature [15] and from proteolysis [16]. The significant difference between the T_c of solutions of proteins isolated from the cortex (2 °C) compared to the nucleus (11–14 °C) at equal concentrations of protein implicates the larger concentration of α-crystallin in the cortex as a stabilizing agent for the phase separation that occurs at low temperature. Our chromatographic data (fig. 4), at concentrations of protein between 2 and 20 mg ml^{-1} provide direct evidence that proteins of the cortex assemble greater quantities of high-molecular-weight protein complexes compared to the nucleus. That α-crystallin has affinity for only heat-denatured γ-crystallin was examined in dilute protein solutions (<1 mg ml^{-1}) [17] in contrast to the experiments we report here for associations between native forms of α- and γ-crystallins. As summarized in figure 5, selenite treatment affects the contributions of protein organization, cellular organization, and the occurrence of low-molecular-weight metabolites as participants in maintaining lens transparency. The model then provides numerous opportunities with which to evaluate intervention in a cataractogenic process.

Acknowledgement

The authors appreciate the excellent technical assistance of Ms. Kathryn Smith, Laboratory Specialist, Department of Biochemistry and Anaerobic Microbiology, Virginia Polytechnic Institute and State University, in handling animals and completing chromatographic separations. This project was supported by NIH grant EY06123.

References

1 Ostadalova I, Babicky A, Obenberger T: Cataract induced by administration of a single dose of sodium selenite to suckling rats. Experientia 1978;34:222–223.
2 Bunce GE, Hess JL: Biochemical changes associated with selenite-induced cataract in the rat. Exp Eye Res 1981;33:505–514.
3 Shearer TR, David LL, Anderson RS: Selenite cataract: A review. Curr Eye Res 1987;6:289–300.
4 David LL, Shearer TR: State of rat lens sulfhydryl groups in selenite cataract. Toxicol Appl Pharmacol 1984;74:109–115.
5 Shearer TR, David LL, Anderson RS: Selenite decreases phase separation temperature in rat lens. Exp Eye Res 1986;42:503–506.
6 Mitton KP, Hess JL, Bunce GE: Causes of decreased phase transition temperature in selenite cataract model. Invest Ophthalmol Vis Sci 1995;36:914–924.
7 Hammer P, Benedek GB: The effect of naturally occurring cellular constituents on phase separation and opacification in calf lens nuclear homogenates. Curr Eye Res 1983;2: 809–814.
8 Bradford MM: A rapid and sensitive method for quantitation of microgram quantities of protein utilizing the principal of protein-dye binding. Anal Biochem 1976;72:248–254.
9 Alder HL, Roessler ES: Introduction to Probability and Statistics, ed 6. San Francisco, Freeman, 1977, pp 330–343.
10 Siezen RJ, Benedek GB: Controlled modulation of the phase separation and opacification temperature of purified bovine γ-IV-crystallin. Curr Eye Res 1983;4:1077–1085.
11 Russell P, Smith SG, Carper DA, Kinoshita JH: Age and cataract related changes in the heavy molecular weight proteins and γ-crystallin composition of the mouse lens. Exp Eye Res 1979;29:245–255.
12 Hiraoka T, Clark JI: Inhibition of lens opacification during the early stages of cataract formation. Invest Ophthalmol Vis Sci 1995;2550–2555.
13 David LL, Wright JW, Shearer TR: Calpain II induced insolubilization of lens β-crystallin polypeptides may induce cataract. Biochim Biophys Acta 1992;1139:210–216.
14 Bunce GE, Hess JL, Batra R: Lens calcium and selenite-induced cataract. Curr Eye Res 1984;3:315–320.
15 Horowitz J: The function of alpha-crystallin. Invest Ophthalmol Vis Sci 1993;43:10–20.
16 Shearer TR, Shih M, Azuma M, David LL: Precipitation of crystallins from young rat lens by endogenous calpain. Exp Eye Res 1995;61: 141–150.
17 Wang K, Spector A: The chaperone activity of bovine α-crystallin: Interaction with other lens crystallins in native and denatured states. J Biol Chem 1994;269:13601–13608.

Ophthalmic Research

Ophthalmic Res 1996;28(suppl 2):54–63

Takashi Hatano
Masami Kojima

Department of Ophthalmology,
Kanazawa Medical University,
Uchinada, Japan

UV-B-Induced Cataract Model in Brown-Norway Rat Eyes Combined with Preadministration of Buthionine Sulfoximine

Key Words
Ultraviolet B
Cataract model
Lens
Brown-Norway rat
Buthionine sulfoximine
Glutathione
Scheimpflug imaging
Image analysis

Abstract
In order to develop a more adequate ultraviolet (UV)-induced cataract model, a combination of *l*-buthionine sulfoximine (BSO) treatment was applied to experimental animals. A single administration of BSO 4 mmol/kg caused reduced glutathione concentration until experimental day 8. In the 0.067-J/cm^2 UV-B irradiation experiment, the light-scattering intensity of the anterior lens cortex of the combination group was significantly higher than that of the other groups during the second week after irradiation commenced. After the fourth experimental week, however, there was no significant difference between the group treated by UV-B alone and the combination group. In the 0.2-J/cm^2 UV-B irradiation experiment, anterior polar cataract was seen in the group receiving UV-B alone, as already reported, 6 weeks after starting UV irradiation. Meanwhile, in the combination group, shallow cortical opacity was seen at 26 weeks after the start of experiment in the deeper lenticular layer which was separated from the anterior subcapsular opacity. This anterior shallow cortical opacity seemed to move towards the nuclear region during the time course of the experiment. The results of this experiment suggested that the BSO treatment accelerated cataractogenesis through additional UV-B irradiation. Although more experiments are needed, this model is useful in investigating the connection between UV-B and other cocataractogenic factors in age-related cataract in humans.

Introduction

In order to investigate the causative factor of human cataract formation, experimental and epidemiological data are principally required. Although the mechanism of age-related cataract formation has not yet been clarified, it may be caused by multiple factors related to the aging process [1–3]. Among these causes, ultraviolet-B (UV-B) irradiation has already been confirmed as a risk factor by a number of basic studies [4–8].

On the other hand, recent worldwide environmental pollution has been considered to be possibly related with depletion of the ozone layer. Consequently, UV irradiation may increase the risk of and induce several UV-caused diseases such as skin cancer or ocular

KARGER

E-Mail karger@karger.ch
Fax + 41 61 306 12 34
http://www.karger.ch

© 1996 S. Karger AG, Basel
0030–3747/96/0288–0054$10.00/0

Takashi Hatano
Department of Ophthalmology
Kanazawa Medical University
Uchinada, Ishikawa 920-02 (Japan)

diseases, including cataract [9]. Therefore, UV-B is again receiving attention as an important physical factor in cataractogenesis today.

UV-B irradiation alone can induce anterior polar cataract in rat eyes in vivo [4–8]. Hockwin et al. [7] reported that when 0.2 J/cm^2 UV-B (every second day) was continuously administered for more than 5 months, opacity initially appeared in the superficial cortical layer and slowly penetrated into the deeper cortex, approaching the supranuclear layer, and posterior opacity along the posterior suture was observed. UV irradiation has been considered a risk for human age-related cataract. However, the type of opacification in the animal model of UV-B-induced cataract is rather different from the types observed in age-related cataract in humans. On the other hand, it is a well-known phenomenon that the cataractous lens has a very low concentration of glutathione. The authors accept both that depression in the lenticular glutathione level is the result of cataract formation and that it accelerates cataract progression, but this is not clear.

In order to clarify the relationship between glutathione depression and cataract progression, the authors' aim was to develop a UV-B-induced cataract model with additional damage to lenticular metabolism. Biochemically compromised rats with partially inhibited glutathione biosynthesis in the lens induced by *l*-buthionine sulfoximine (BSO) were used as experimental animals.

Materials and Methods

Administration of BSO and Determination of Glutathione

A total of 36 male 8-week-old Brown-Norway rats were divided into two groups of 18 rats each. One, 2, 4, 8, 16, and 32 days after a single intraperitoneal injection of BSO at 4 mmol/kg (Sigma), 6 eyes of 3 rats were removed after an intravenously injected overdose of pentobarbital sodium and the lenses dissected from the eyeballs, after which the lenses were immediately frozen at –70 °C for 2 h. Then the lens was divided into 4 pieces; the equator, the anterior cortex, the nucleus and the posterior cortex to prepare for microsectioning analysis [5, 10] (fig. 1). The same samples from 6 lenses of 3 non-BSO-treated rats were prepared as controls. Nonprotein SH, as the total glutathione concentration of each lens layers, was measured by the DTNB method [11]: The lens layers were weighed and homogenized in ice-cold distilled water (1:9 w/v). After centrifuging (at 12,000 *g* for 10 min 0 °C), a 1% picric acid solution (5 v/v of homogenate) was added for protein denaturation. The glutathione concentration in the supernatant was measured as follows: an NADPH/buffer solution, DTNB solution, and sample were placed in the cuvette. The reaction was started by pipetting a glutathione reductase solution into the cuvette and immediately placing it in the spectrophotometer. The glutathione concentration was measured by monitoring the absorbance decrease of NADPH at 412 nm for 4 min. Glutathione concentration in the samples was calculated by $\Delta A \cdot min^{-1}$.

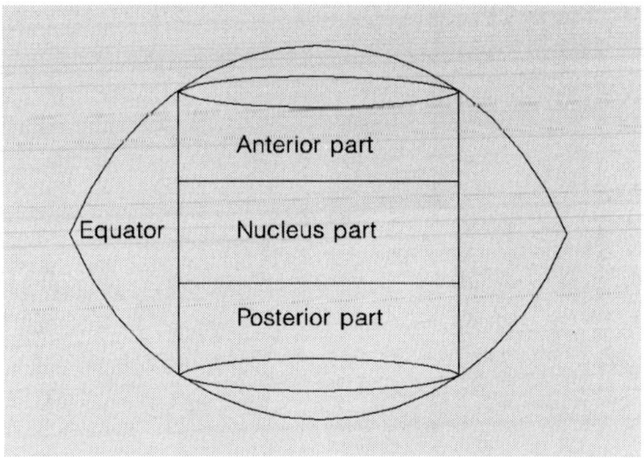

Fig. 1. The division of frozen lenses with the lens-sectioning method: The lens is divided into the cylinder and equatorial part with the cylinder diameter representing 80% of the lens diameter. The cylinder was divided into 3 parts with the same thickness.

UV-B Irradiation

Thirty-two male 10-week-old Brown-Norway rats were divided into four groups of 8 rats each (table 1): Group 1-A (Gr. 1-A) received no treatment (normal control group). Group 2-A (Gr. 2-A) received a single

Table 1. Grouping of rats

Group	n	No treatment	BSO	UV low	UV high
1-A	8	*			
1-B	6	*			
2-A	8		*		
2-B	6		*		
3-A	8			*	
3-B	6				*
4-A	8		*	*	
4-B	6		*		*

intraperitoneal administration of BSO at 4 mmol/kg. Group 3-A (Gr. 3-A) received a UV-B irradiation dose of 0.067 J/cm^2 once a week for 20 weeks continuously with a total dose of 1.34 J/cm^2. Group 4-A (Gr. 4-A) rats were administered BSO in the same way as Gr. 2-A rats and were irradiated with UV as Gr. 3-A. UV-B irradiation was performed with a 20-watt UV-B lamp (Orion Ltd. FL20S-E-30, peak wave length 310 nm, range 265–400 nm) attached to an instrument for psoralen UV-A therapy (Orion, OR-114). Pupils were dilated with a topical 1% atropine sulfate solution. Eighty percent of the irradiation wavelength was 310 nm.

Twenty-four male 10-week-old Brown-Norway rats were divided into four groups of 6 rats each (table 1): Gr. 1-B received no treatment (normal control), Gr. 2-B received a single intraperitoneal administration of BSO 4 mmol/kg, Gr. 3-B was irradiated with 0.2 J/cm^2 of UV-B, every other day for 2 weeks, and Gr. 4-B received a single intraperitoneal administration of 4 mmol/kg before UV-B irradiation of 0.2 J/cm^2 every other day for 2 weeks. The total UV irradiation dose for Gr. 3-B and Gr. 4-B was 1.6 J/cm^2.

Observation and Documentation of Lenticular Changes

Changes in lenticular transparency were observed by slit-lamp microscopy and documented by an anterior eye segment analysis system (EAS-1000, NIDEK) [12, 13] with pupils dilated by instillation of a 0.5% tropicamide and 0.5% phenylephrine mixture (Mydrin P®, Santen). Image analysis was performed by software integrated in the system, which was developed by Sasaki et al. [12].

Results

Changes of Glutathione Levels after Intraperitoneal BSO Administration in Lenses

Total glutathione concentrations in the lenses were examined in each separated lens section. One day after BSO administration, the total glutathione concentration of the anterior and posterior layers had significantly decreased compared with that of the control lenses, whereas the equatorial region showed only a tendency to decrease. On the second day, the area of significant decrease in glutathione concentration spread to the anterior, posterior, and equatorial regions. On the fourth day, glutathione concentration in the anterior and posterior parts of the lenses showed a tendency to return to the normal level; however, that in the equatorial region was still significantly lower than that of the control lenses. On the eighth day, the concentrations of glutathione in the posterior and equatorial regions were still significantly low. On the sixteenth and thirty-second days, no significant differences of glutathione concentration between the lenses of the control and those of the BSO-treated groups were left. The glutathione levels in the nuclei of both the BSO-treated and nontreated groups were stable throughout the experiment (table 2); figure 2 demonstrates more clearly the changes in glutathione concentration with the time course.

Changes in Lenticular Transparency after Low-Dose UV-B Irradiation Combined with BSO Administration

No marked corneal damage such as erosion, edema or opacification which could disturb the observation of lenticular changes was noticed after irradiation with a 0.067 J/cm^2 UV-B dose. Light-scattering intensity in the lenses of both control and BSO-treated rats

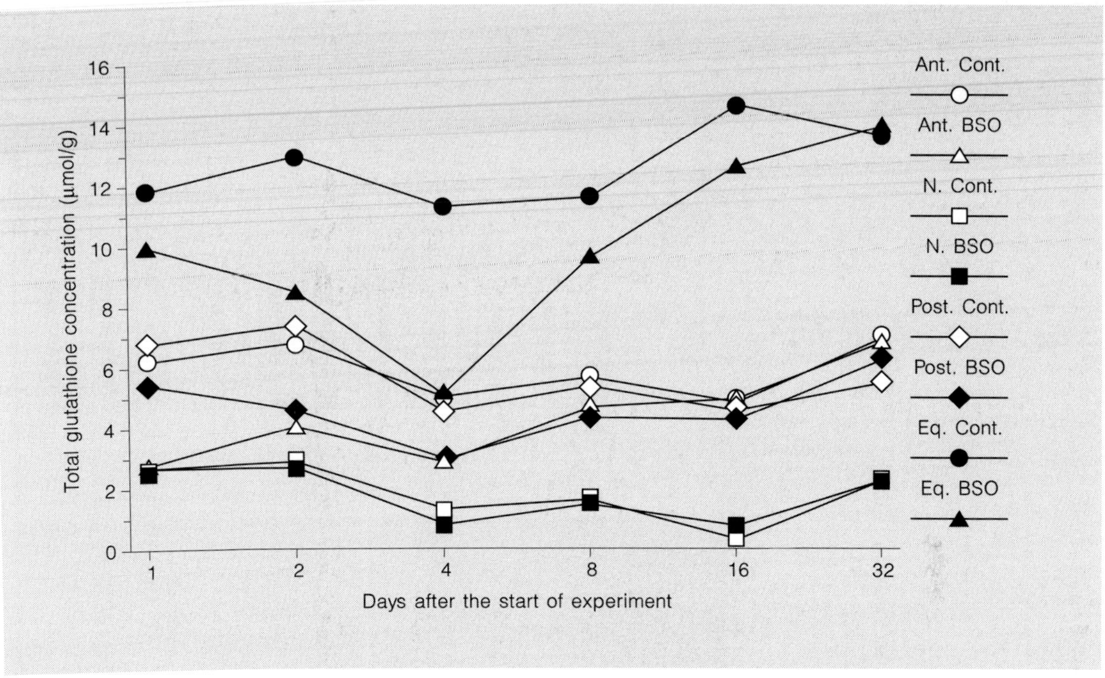

Fig. 2. Changes in mean values of total glutathione in each of the 4 parts with the course of time. For further explanations see table 1. Ant. = Anterior cortex; Cont. = control lenses; BSO = BSO-treated lenses; N. = nucleus; Post = posterior cortex; Eq. = equator.

Table 2. Mean values (± SD) of total glutathione concentration (µmol/g) in each of the 4 parts of the lenses (n = 6), measured on days 1, 2, 4, 8, 16 and 32 after beginning the experiment

	Day 1	Day 2	Day 4	Day 8	Day 16	Day 32
Ant.						
Cont.	6.2±0.2 ┐*	6.8±0.5 ┐**	5.0±1.3	5.7±0.3	4.8±0.4	7.1±0.8
BSO	2.7±1.1 ┘	4.1±0.6 ┘	2.9±1.5	4.7±0.7	4.9±1.2	6.9±1.0
N.						
Cont.	2.6±0.4	2.9±0.2	1.3±0.1	1.7±0.2	0.3±0.2	2.3±0.2
BSO	2.7±0.6	2.7±0.3	0.8±0.4	1.5±0.1	0.8±0.5	2.3±0.1
Post.						
Cont.	6.7±0.5 ┐*	7.4±0.8 ┐*	4.6±0.5	5.4±0.0 ┐**	4.6±0.1	5.6±0.2
BSO	5.4±0.3 ┘	4.6±0.7 ┘	3.0±1.9	4.3±0.1 ┘	4.3±1.0	6.4±0.6
Eq.						
Cont.	11.8±1.0	13.0±1.8 ┐*	11.3±0.8 ┐**	11.6±0.7 ┐*	14.7±2.1	13.7±1.0
BSO	10.0±2.6	8.5±0.4 ┘	5.1±1.5 ┘	9.7±0.2 ┘	12.7±2.6	14.0±2.9

* $p < 0.05$; ** $p < 0.01$. Ant. = Anterior cortex; Cont. = control lenses; N = nucleus; Post. = posterior cortex; Eq. = equator; BSO = BSO-treated lenses.

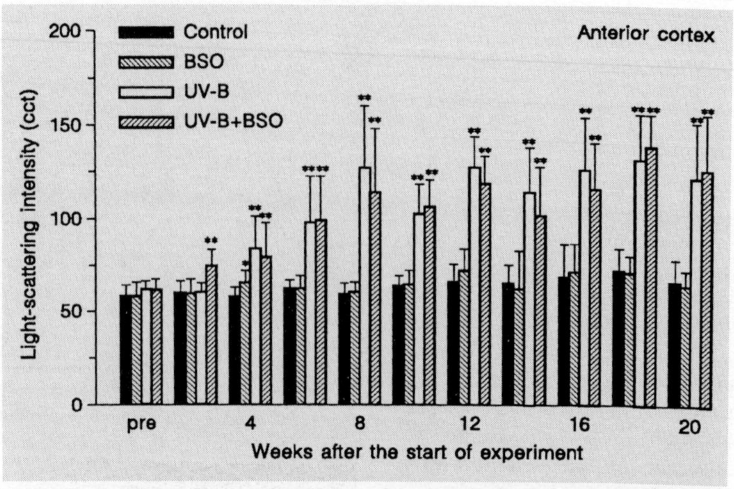

Fig. 3. Mean values (± SD) of densitometric peak heights of the anterior cortex in all four groups with the dose of 0.067 J/cm² UV-B. * $p < 0.05$, ** $p < 0.01$, controls vs. treatment group.

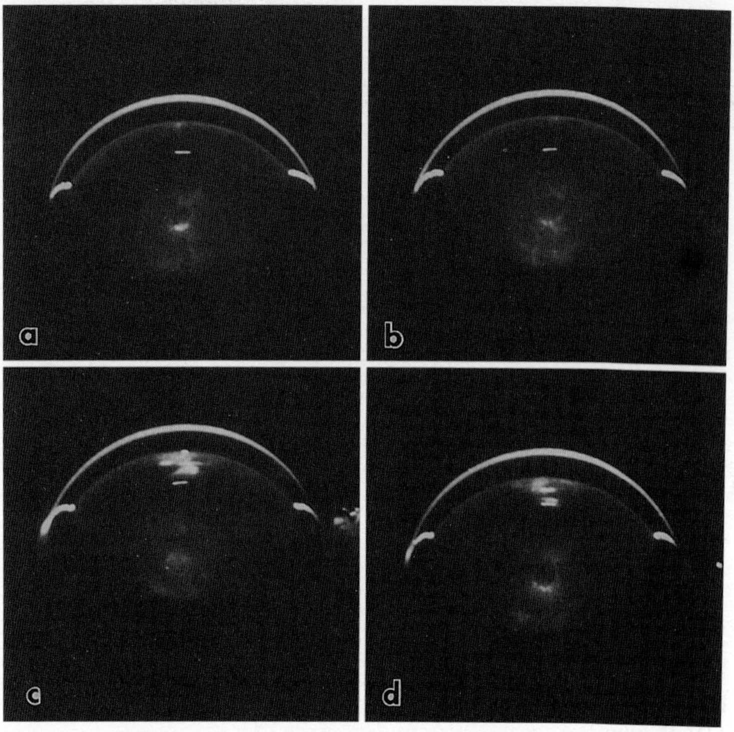

Fig. 4. Scheimpflug images of each of the four groups 20 weeks after the 0.067-J/cm² UV-B treatment. The normal controls (**a**) and the BSO-treated group (**b**) showed no cataractous change. A UV-B dose of 0.067 J/cm² without BSO (**c**) and a combination of UV-B and BSO administration (**d**) demonstrated progressive anterior cortical opacity.

remained almost stable during the experimental period. There was no difference in the light-scattering intensity of lenticular layers between the controls and the group treated with BSO alone. Two weeks after the beginning of UV-B irradiation, the light-scattering intensity of the anterior shallow cortex region of the rats in Gr. 4-A was significantly higher than that of the other groups (Gr. 1-A, Gr. 2-A, and Gr. 3-A). Four weeks after the start of

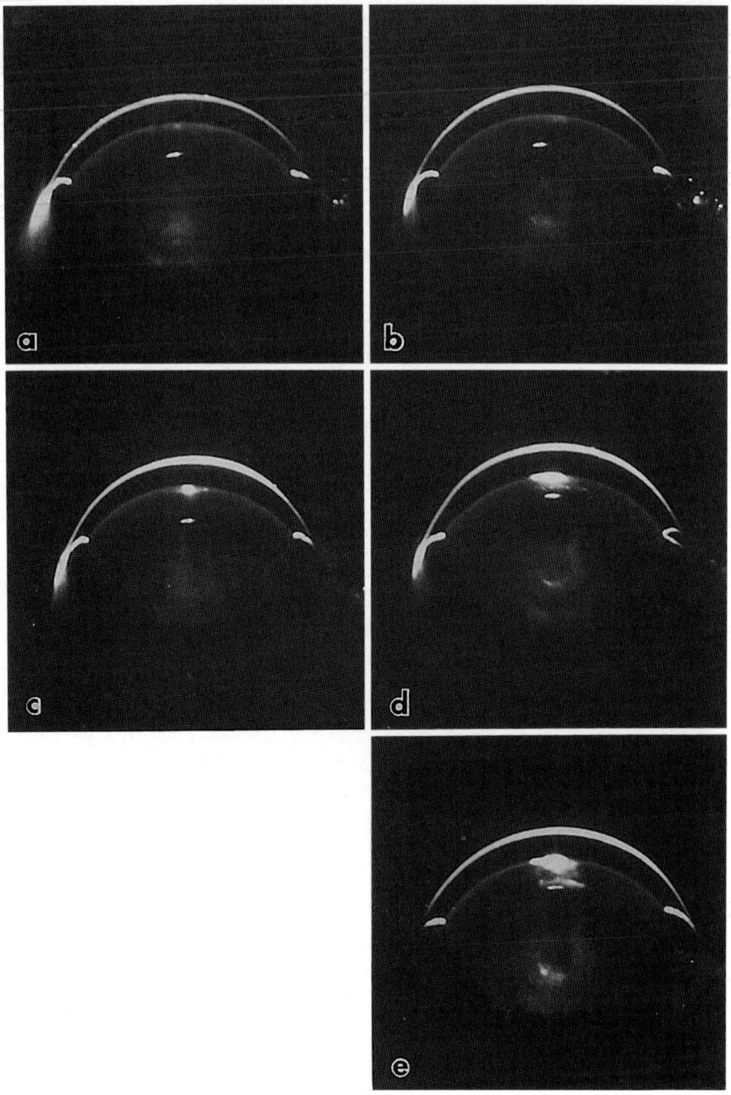

Fig. 5. Scheimpflug images of each of the four groups 6 weeks after starting the 0.2-J/cm^2 UV-B treatment. The normal control (**a**) and BSO-treated (**b**) groups showed no lens opacification. The group treated with 0.2 J/cm^2 UV-B (**c**) showed anterior subcapsular cataracts. The combination group (**d**) demonstrated strong light-scattering intensity at the anterior subcapsular and shallow cortical region. The photograph (**e**) demonstrates the lens condition 26 weeks after treatment in the combination group. The shallow cortical opacity appeared deeper than at 6 weeks (**d**).

UV-B irradiation, the light-scattering intensity at the same place in the group treated by UV-B irradiation alone (Gr. 3-A) and the combination group (Gr. 4-A) was significantly higher than that seen in the controls (Gr. 1-A) and the group treated by BSO (Gr. 2-A) alone (fig. 3). The anterior subcapsular opacity of rats in Gr. 3-A and Gr. 4-A extended to the anterior shallow cortical layer, and continued to progress toward the nuclear area in both groups until the end of the 20-week observation period (fig. 4a–d).

Changes in Lenticular Transparency after High-Dose UV-B Irradiation in Combination with BSO Administration

No prominent lenticular alterations were observed in the controls (Gr. 1-B) or Gr. 2-B (receiving only BSO, fig. 5a, b). Six weeks after beginning UV irradiation, lenticular changes were noticed in the limited area of the anterior subcapsular region in Gr. 3-B (fig. 5c), while in Gr. 4-B, initial lens changes appeared in the anterior subcapsular and anterior shallow cortical regions. The above opacifications were noticed 6 weeks after the initial irradiation. The area of the anterior opacity was larger in Gr. 4-B than in Gr. 3-B. No precise observation of the lens was possible until 5 weeks after starting UV irradiation, due to a hazy cornea. The anterior subcapsular opacity in rats in Gr. 3-B showed no remarkable changes and stayed in the same area up to 26 weeks after the initial UV-B irradiation. The lens opacification in the anterior shallow cortical layer in Gr. 4-B moved toward the nuclear region with the course of time. After 26 weeks, two types of opacity were observed: anterior subcapsular and cortical opacities (fig. 5d, e), which were completely separate from each other. The movement of the cortical opacities towards the deeper region showed a constant progression ratio (fig. 6a, b).

Discussion

Among the risk factors related to human cataract formation, UV-B has been considered a possible causative factor [1–3, 9]. Although experimental proof has been offered by previous authors [4–8], it is still difficult to conclude that UV-B alone is causative in the formation of age-related cataract in humans.

The authors accept without doubt the multifactorial pathogenesis of human cataracts with a combination of syn- and/or cocataractogenic risk factors [14]. In fact, UV irradiation has often been applied to experimentally induced cataract as additional damage [15–17]. Therefore the authors have considered that UV-B radiation may correlate with the acceleration of cataract formation or progression together with other cocataractogenic factors.

As described in the introduction, recent epidemiological studies of UV-related cataracts [1–3] again require further basic data concerning cataracts induced purely by UV-B; this in turn would require a more complex experimental model, which led us to attempt a new type of UV-B-induced cataract using an animal model.

According to the investigation by Calvin et al. [18], it was possible to induce the state of nearly total depletion of glutathione in the lenses of suckling mice by repeated administration of BSO at 4 mmol/kg. Since it is well known that glutathione levels are reduced in cataractous lenses [19, 20], the authors applied the phenomenon induced by systemic BSO administration to UV-B-induced experimental cataract. Intraperitoneal administration of BSO at 4 mmol/kg in Brown-Norway rats induced a moderate reduction of glutathione in the lens, especially in the anterior cortical and equatorial parts, but only for a period of 1 week.

With the purpose of inducing a glutathione-depleted state, 2 different doses of UV-B irradiation were used. The dose of 0.2 J/cm^2 irradiation induced severe corneal damage, as reported by previous authors [4, 7, 8]. On the other hand, no corneal damage was induced with a dose of 0.067 J/cm^2.

A comparison of the corneal and lenticular changes observed in subjects undergoing different doses of UV-B irradiation combined with BSO administration revealed the following: a low dose of UV-B (0.067 J/cm^2) in the non-BSO-treated group showed that anterior cortical opacity had progressed toward the deeper cortex during the experimental period. Although the authors had expected that the combination of UV radiation and BSO treatment might accelerate cataract progression and/or severity, there was no prominent dif-

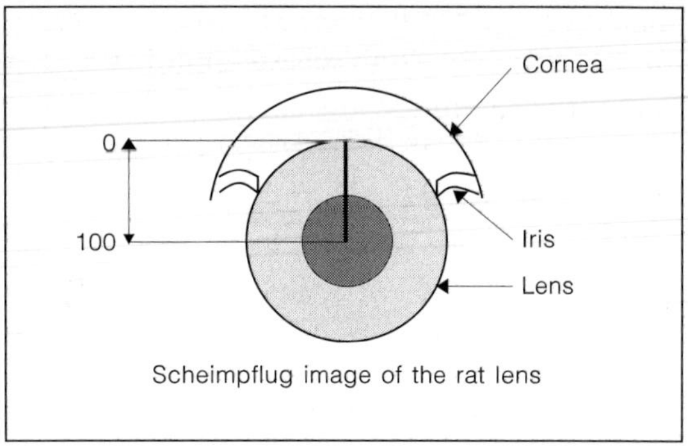

a

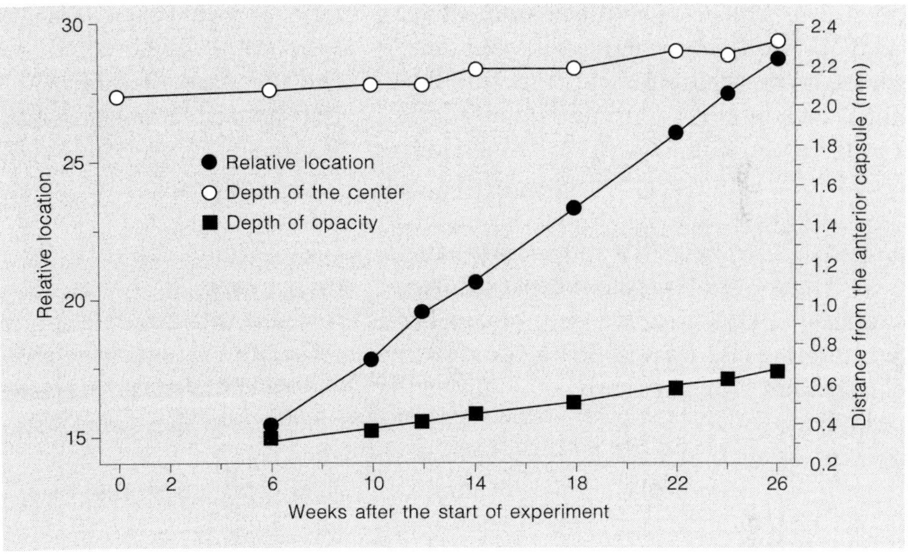

b

Fig. 6. A schema of lens opacity movement. **a** Definition of relative location of opacity. **b** Alterations of the biometrical results and relative location.

ference between the rats with the combined UV and BSO treatment and rats with UV irradiation alone. Only a small accelerative effect, which might be related with the formation of lens opacification, was noticed. The UV-B and BSO combination group rats (Gr. 4-A) showed a significantly higher light-scattering intensity compared with the other three groups, 2 weeks after the start of the experiment (fig. 3). A possible reason for the above phenomenon would be that a single BSO administration led to a decrease in the glutathione level of the lens for only 1 week, creating no significant difference between UV-B treatment alone (Gr. 3-A) and combined UV-B and BSO treatment from 4 weeks after the start of the experiment.

Precise observation of rat lenses that had received a high dose of UV irradiation during the first 5 weeks could not be performed due to a hazy cornea, which gradually disappeared after 6 weeks. Cortical opacity was seen during 6 weeks. Although light-scattering intensity was higher and the opaque area was larger in the high-dose UV irradiation group than in the low-dose UV irradiation group, there was no prominent difference in lens opacification. Although the results obtained were interesting, and have not been reported before, it is still unclear whether different susceptibilities exist in the lens to chronic low doses of UV irradiation and acute high doses of UV irradiation.

In the group with combined administration, two types of opacification were observed: anterior polar and shallow cortical opacities, and cortical opacity. These two opacities, located in different layers, were separated by normal lenticular fibers both macroscopically and photographically. There have been several reports that the anterior subcapsular opacity slowly penetrates into the deeper cortex, approaching the supranuclear layer, under long-term UV-B irradiation to rats [6–8]. One of the authors performed a long-term (156 day) UV-B irradiation study with a high dose (0.2 J/cm^2) and low dose (0.15 J/cm^2) in an early experiment [8], and found that the peak heights and the peak bases of anterior subcapsular opacification were enlarged on Scheimpflug lens images. The reason for the enlargement of the opaque area might be the destruction of the lenticular fibers such as swelling or disruption of the fibers as well as liquefaction extending to the neighboring lenticular fibers. In contrast, two distinct kinds of opacification were observed in this experiment. To explain these findings, two actions are possible: First, since UV-B irradiation was performed for only 2 weeks, newly synthesized normal transparent lenticular fibers might appear beneath the epithelium after the interruption of UV-B irradiation. The other possibility is that the depression of glutathione by BSO was only induced for 1 week, and newly synthesized lenticular fibers pushed the affected fibers toward the deeper layer after the concentration of glutathione returned to a normal level.

In spite of interrupting UV radiation 2 weeks after the start of the experiment, anterior subcapsular opacification was still observed 26 weeks later. The reason for this phenomenon is unclear. However, Hightower et al. [21] reported that a primary target of UV-B irradiation in the crystalline lens is the lenticular epithelium. If so, the continuous progression of opacification for a certain period might occur. Almost all UV radiation below 290 nm is absorbed by the corneal layer. Hyperplasia of the lenticular epithelial cells [8] in UV-exposed lenses might be an absorbing barrier for the further penetration of UV radiation into the deeper lenticular layers. The movement of anterior cortical opacity area toward the nuclear region that was observed in the investigation had the same appearance as that seen in the UV-induced cataract in a human case reported by Mueller-Breitenkamp et al. [22].

An unexpected result was that results of the combination treatment group with low UV-B irradiation (0.067 J/cm^2) and glutathione depression were not prominently different from those of the group receiving UV-B alone. The authors were able to induce rather prominent cortical cataracts without corneal damage in the group treated with UV-B alone.

Several questions regarding experimentally induced UV-related cataracts remain. However, the experimental cataract model induced by UV irradiation with BSO administration may become a suitable model to investigate the formation of anterior cortical cataracts.

Acknowledgments

The authors are grateful for the grants 'The Influence of UV-B Radiation on Human Health' from the Environmental Agency of Japan. The authors thank Prof. K. Sasaki (Department of Ophthalmology) for the helpful discussion, advice, and guidance. The valuable advice and revision of the manuscript by Prof. Dr. O. Hockwin, Guest professor of Kanazawa Medical University, Prof. Y. Kawarai (Second Department of Anatomy), and Prof. S. Imanishi (Second Department of Physiology) are gratefully appreciated.

References

1 Taylor HR, West SK, Rosenthal FS, Munoz B, Newland HS, Abbey H, Emmett EA: Effect of ultraviolet radiation on cataract formation. N Engl J Med 1988;319:1429–1433.

2 Hu T, Lao Y: An epidemiologic survey of senile cataract in China; in Sasaki K, Hockwin O, Leske MC (eds): Cataract Epidemiology. Dev Ophthalmol. Basel, Karger, 1987, vol 15, pp 42–51.

3 Rink H: Cataractogenic risk factors; in Sasaki K, Hockwin O, Leske MC (eds): Cataract Epidemiology. Dev Ophthalmol. Basel, Karger, 1987, vol 15, pp 66–76.

4 Wegener A, Hockwin O: Animal models as a tool to detect the subliminal cocataractogenic potential of drugs; in Hockwin O (ed): Drug-Induced Ocular Side Effects and Ocular Toxicology. Basel, Karger, 1987, pp 250–262.

5 Kojima M: Regional enzymatic analysis of UV-B and streptozotocin induced diabetic cataract lens. Lens Eye Toxicol Res 1990;7:547–561.

6 Schmidt J, Schmitt C, Wegener A, Hockwin O: Histological changes of rat lenses after UV-irradiation and *D*-penicillamine treatment. Ophthalmic Res 1993;25:69–76.

7 Hockwin O, Wegener A, Bessems G, Bours J, Korte I, Mueller-Breitenkamp U, Schmidt J, Schmitt C: Models and methods for testing toxicity: Lens; in Hockwin O, Green K, Rubin LF (eds): Manual of Oculotoxicity Testing of Drugs. Stuttgart, Gustav Fischer, 1992, pp 255–316.

8 Schmidt J, Schmitt C, Kojima M, Hockwin O: Biochemical and morphological changes in rat lenses after long-term UV B irradiation. Ophthalmic Res 1992;24:317–325.

9 World Health Organization: INTERSUN: A Global UV Project, Protection against Exposure to Ultraviolet Radiation. Geneva, WHO, 1995.

10 Mueller A, Moeller B, Dragomirescu V, Hockwin O: Profiles of enzyme activities in bovine lenses; in Hockwin O (ed): Drug-Induced Ocular Side Effects and Ocular Toxicology. Basel, Karger, 1987, pp 343–349.

11 Griffith OW: Glutathione and glutathione disulphide; in Bergmeyer HU (ed): Methods of Enzymatic Analysis. Weinheim, VCH Publishers, 1985, vol 8, pp 521–529.

12 Sasaki K, Sakamoto Y, Shibata T, Emori Y: The multi-purpose camera: A new anterior eye segment analysis system. Ophthalmic Res 1990;22(suppl 1):3–8.

13 Kojima M, Sasaki K: Application of a new Scheimpflug camera (EAS-1000) to animal cataract models. Ophthalmic Res 1992;24(suppl 1): 3–9.

14 Hockwin O, Wegener A: Syn- and cocataractogenesis – A system for testing subliminal lens toxicity; in Hockwin O (ed): Drug-Induced Ocular Side Effects and Ocular Toxicology. Basel, Karger, 1987, pp 241–249.

15 Schmidt J, Brettner S, Wegener A, Hockwin O: Ultraviolet-induced changes in corneal transmission properties and influence on Scheimpflug photography. Ophthalmic Res 1990;22:365–370.

16 Breadsell RO, Wegener A, Breipohl W, Hirst LW: UV-B radiation-induced cataract in the Royal College of Surgeons rat. Ophthalmic Res 1994;26(suppl 1):84–89.

17 Malik A, Kojima M, Sasaki K: Morphological and biochemical changes in lenses of guinea pigs after vitamin-C-deficient diet and UV-B radiation. Ophthalmic Res 1995;27: 189–196.

18 Calvin HI, Hagen SV, Hess JL, Patel SA, Fu SCJ: Lens GSH depletion and electrolyte changes preceding cataracts induced by buthionine sulfoximine in suckling mice. Exp Eye Res 1992;54:621–626.

19 Pau H, Graf P, Sies H: Glutathione levels in human lenses: Regional distribution in different forms of cataract. Exp Eye Res 1990;50:17–20.

20 Chakrapani B, Yedavally S, Leverenz V, Goblin FJ, Reddy VN: Simultaneous measurement of reduced and oxidized glutathione in human aqueous humor and cataracts by electrochemical detection. Ophthalmic Res 1995;27(suppl 1): 69–77.

21 Hightower KR, Reddan JR, McCready JP, Dziedzic DC: Lens epithelium: A primary target of UVB irradiation. Exp Eye Res 1994; 59:557–564.

22 Mueller-Breitenkamp U, Hockwin O, Siekmann H, Dragomirescu V: Ultraviolet radiation as cataract risk factor – A case report. Dev Ophthalmol. Basel, Karger, 1996 (in press).

Ophthalmic Research

Ophthalmic Res 1996;28(suppl 2):64–71

Masami Kojima
Ying Bo Shui
Hidekazu Murano
Kazuyuki Sasaki

Department of Ophthalmology,
Kanazawa Medical University,
Uchinada, Ishikawa, Japan

Inhibition of Steroid-Induced Cataract in Rat Eyes by Administration of Vitamin-E Ophthalmic Solution

Key Words
Lens
Steroid-induced cataract
Vitamin-E ophthalmic solution
Drug efficacy
Brown Norway rat

Abstract
The efficacy of a vitamin-E (VE) ophthalmic solution was evaluated on a newly developed rat steroid-induced cataract model. Brown Norway rats irradiated with 2 Gy X-ray, right eyes only, were divided into 5 groups: the control group; 2 steroid (1 mg/kg/day)-treated groups with topic (Top) and systemic (Sys) administration, and 2 VE-treated groups, 1 with the same treatment as the Top group with the addition of 5% VE twice a day (Top + VE) and 1 with the same treatment as the Sys group with 5% VE twice a day (SYS + VE). The lens changes were documented with a Scheimpflug camera and changes in light scattering were evaluated quantitatively. The VE-treated groups (Top + VE and Sys + VE) showed a significant inhibition of the increase in the opaque area compared with each of the non-VE-treated groups. The VE ophthalmic solution was strong enough to prevent steroid-induced cataract in rats.

Introduction

Corticosteroids are very powerful when administered both systemically and topically to treat inflammatory and immune disorders, and have therefore been widely prescribed clinically. On the other hand, since the report of Black et al. [1] in 1960 of a high incidence of posterior subcapsular cataract in 44 patients with rheumatoid arthritis, many studies concerning steroid-induced posterior subcapsular cataract have been performed. The corticosteroid-induced cataract was fully reviewed by Urban and Cotlier [2] in 1986. With no suitable animal model for steroid-induced cataract [3] up to now, there has been no adequate therapy besides cataract surgery.

KARGER

E-Mail karger@karger.ch
Fax + 41 61 306 12 34
http://www.karger.ch

© 1996 S. Karger AG, Basel
0030–3747/96/0288–0064$10.00/0

Masami Kojima, PhD
1-1, Daigaku
Uchinada-machi
Kahoku-gun
Ishikawa 920-02 (Japan)

Since steroid treatment is often long-term, safety is an important aspect when looking for drug therapy for steroid-induced cataract. Nutrients such as vitamin C (ascorbate), vitamin E (VE, α-tocopherol) and carotenoids have been thought to be relatively safe with respect to overdosing. A recent epidemiological case-control study showed that the risk for cataract development was reduced to one half in the lenses of persons with higher levels of VE [4]. In general, oral administration of the above-mentioned nutrients penetrates very little into the eye, especially when the pharmacological target is the crystalline lens. Moreover, to reduce the side effects of long-term drug therapy and to achieve a sufficient drug concentration to penetrate the lens, topical administration is more effective than systemic administration.

Recently we successfully developed a steroid-induced posterior cataract model in rats [5]. This experiment was designed to evaluate the efficacy of a VE ophthalmic solution for steroid-induced cataract in rats.

Materials and Methods

Six-week-old male Brown Norway rats were used as experimental animals. Two weeks before steroid administration, the right eyes of all animals received a single 2-Gy dose of X-ray irradiation as a subliminal cataract induction dose, while the entire animal body including the left eye was protected. Details of the experimental procedure have been reported previously [5]. X-Irradiated rats were divided into 5 groups. Six rats without drug administration served as controls; 9 rats in the topical eye drop group (Top) were instilled with 1% prednisolone acetate (1 mg/kg/day) ophthalmic solutions in both eyes, and 12 rats in the systemic group (Sys) received a 0.8- to 1.0-mg/kg/day prednisolone acetate injection into the muscle. Of the 2 VE groups, 1 group underwent the same treatment as the Top group with the addition of a 5% VE ophthalmic solution (Santen Pharmaceutical Co., Ltd.) administered into both eyes twice a day (Top + VE, 8 rats), and the other group received the same treatment as the Sys group with the same 5% VE administration (Sys + VE, 12 rats; table 1). Steroid administration was performed in the morning and VE was instilled in the afternoon.

Table 1. Treatment of the 5 groups

Group	n	Topical VE, %	Prednisolone mg/kg/day	
			topical	systemic
Control	6	0	0	0
Top	9	0	1	0
Sys	12	0	0	0.8–1.0
Top + VE	8	5	1	0
Sys + VE	12	5	0	0.8–1.0

Rat lenses were examined by slit lamp microscopy and documented with a Scheimpflug camera (EAS-1000, NIDEK) [6, 7] in maximal mydriasis (0.5% phenylephrine and 0.5% tropicamide solution, Midrin P®) before the start of the experiment and once a month after the start of prednisolone administration. The body weight and blood glucose levels of the rats were checked as general health conditions once a week and every 2 weeks, respectively. Blood glucose levels were measured using a glucose oxidase method (Glutest E®, Sanwa) under nonfasting conditions.

Changes in lens transparency were evaluated by applying a modified program for opaque area measurement of retroillumination cataract images. The first step was to evaluate Scheimpflug slit images utilizing a circle mask which did not overlap the images of the cornea or iris. The second step was to measure the area of corneal reflex. In the third step, the total pixels of the encircled area, including corneal reflex area, were measured. In the fourth step, the true opaque area was elaborated by calculating the total pixels obtained from step 3 minus the corneal pixels from step 2 [5].

Results

General Health Conditions

The body weight of the control group which received 2 Gy X-ray irradiation increased from 177 ± 11 g at the start of the experiment to 377 ± 22 g 50 weeks later. This body weight gain of the control group did not differ from that of the nonirradiated animals.

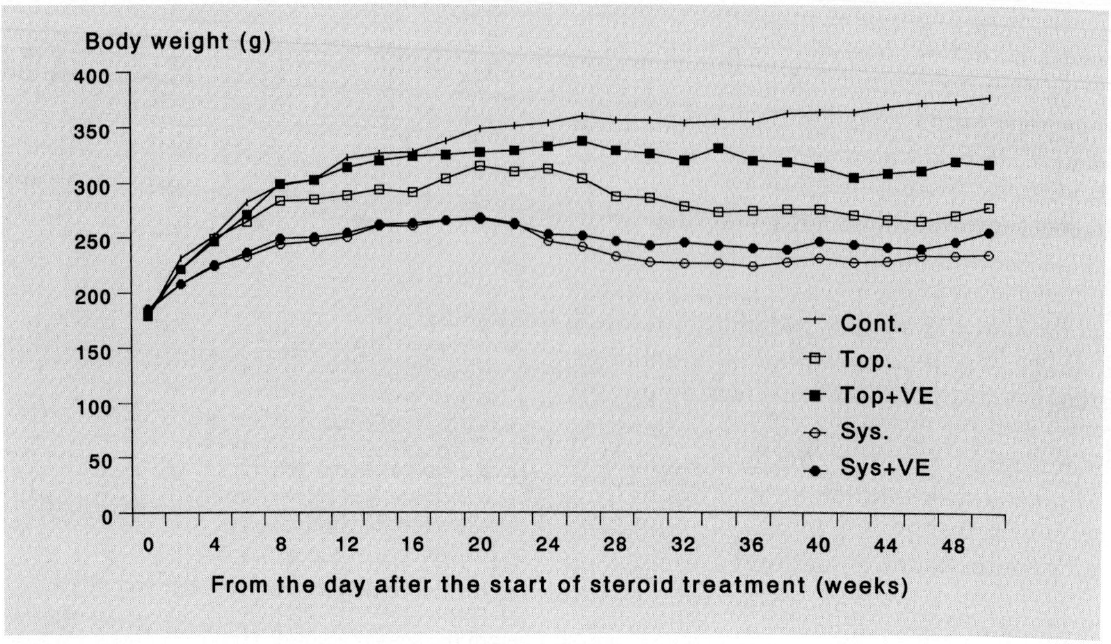

Fig. 1. Body weight fluctuation in the 5 experimental groups.

The body weights of the Top group increased from 183 ± 9 to 304 ± 25 g. A significant difference in body weight gain was found between the control and Top groups 11 weeks after the start of steroid treatment. The Sys group showed the lowest body weight gain of the 5 groups (initial 185 ± 8 and final 268 ± 17 g). A significant difference in body weight was found between the Sys and Control groups 1 week after the start of the experiment. The body weight gains of the Top + VE and Sys + VE groups were slightly higher than those of the Top and Sys groups (fig. 1).

The blood glucose fluctuation of the 5 groups was in the 67- to 97-mg/dl range throughout the experimental period. Although the systemically administered steroid groups (Sys and Sys + VE) showed a blood glucose increase from the 11th to the 30th weeks compared with the control group ($p < 0.05$), it was only a slight difference and not in the range of diabetes.

Changes in Lens Transparency Evaluated by Slit Lamp Examination

No prominent changes in lens transparency were seen in the control group during the 1-year experimental period. The Top group developed anterior cortical and posterior subcapsular opacification in both the X-ray-irradiated and nonirradiated eyes. Meanwhile, the Sys group showed anterior cortical opacity and some rats developed posterior subcapsular cataract. In contrast, the Top + VE group developed a slight cortical opacity on the X-ray-irradiated right eyes, but not on the nonirradiated left eyes. The Sys + VE showed slight anterior cortical changes on the irradiated right eyes, but no prominent lens changes in the nonirradiated left eyes at the end of the experiment (fig. 2, 3).

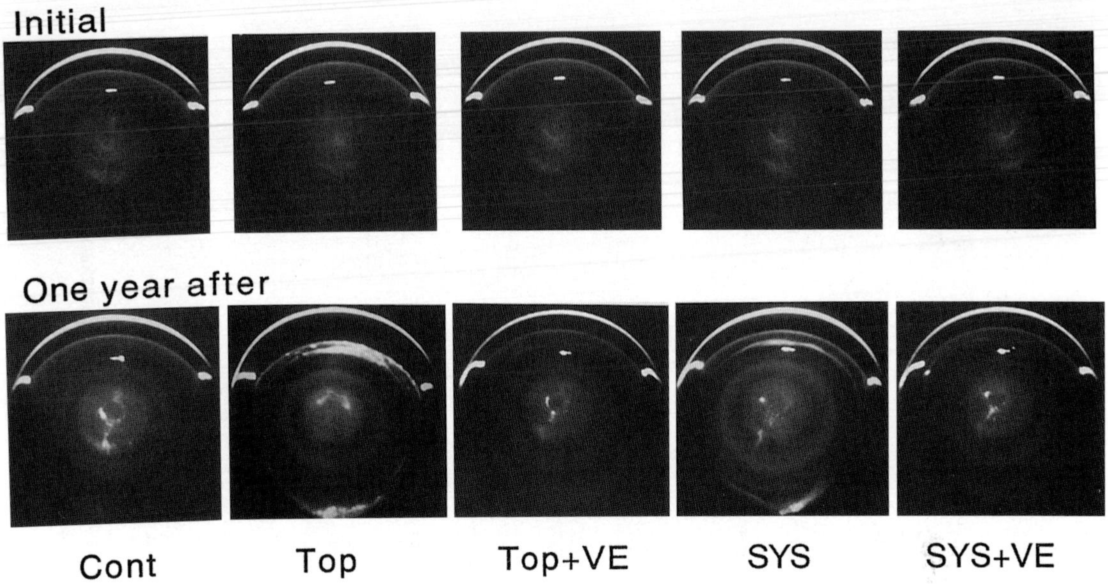

Fig. 2. Representative lens conditions in the X-ray-irradiated right eyes initially and 1 year after the start of the experiment in the 5 groups.

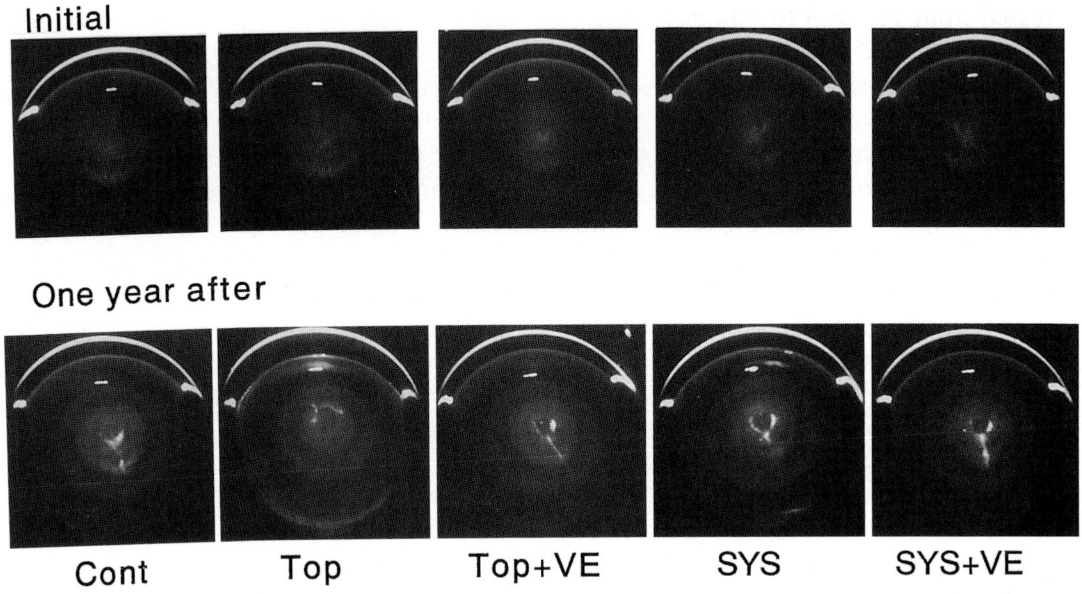

Fig. 3. Representative lens condition in the non-X-ray-irradiated left eyes initially and 1 year after the start of the experiment in the 5 groups.

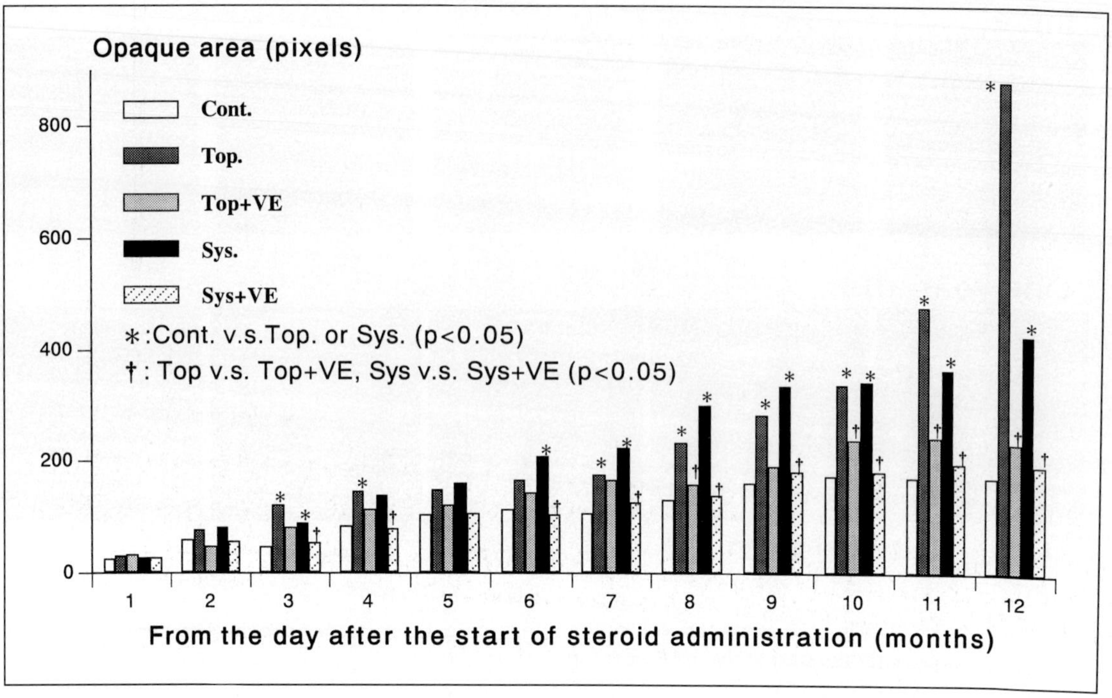

Fig. 4. Opaque area changes in X-ray-irradiated right eyes during the 1-year experimental period in the 5 groups.

Changes in Lens Opacity Seen through Image Analysis

X-Irradiated Right Eyes. The control group (no steroid administration) showed a slight increase in light scattering intensity throughout the whole examination period (fig. 4). The Top group showed a significant increase (except in the 5th month) in opaque area 9 months after the start of steroid administration. The Top + VE group also showed a gradual increase in the opaque area; however, the lens changes were significantly reduced in comparison with the Top group 10 months after the start of VE treatment. The Sys group showed a significant increase in the opaque area 6 months after the start of the experiment. In contrast, the opaque area of the Sys + VE group was always smaller than that of the Sys group and a statistical difference was observed from the 3rd to the 12th month (except in the 5th month).

Nonirradiated Left Eyes. Changes in the opaque areas of the left lenses in the 5 experimental groups were almost the same as those of the irradiated right lenses (fig. 5). Again, the Top + VE and Sys + VE groups showed a significant delay in the increase in opaque area compared with the Top and Sys groups not given VE.

The opaque area of the irradiated right lenses was a bit larger than that of the nonirradiated left lenses.

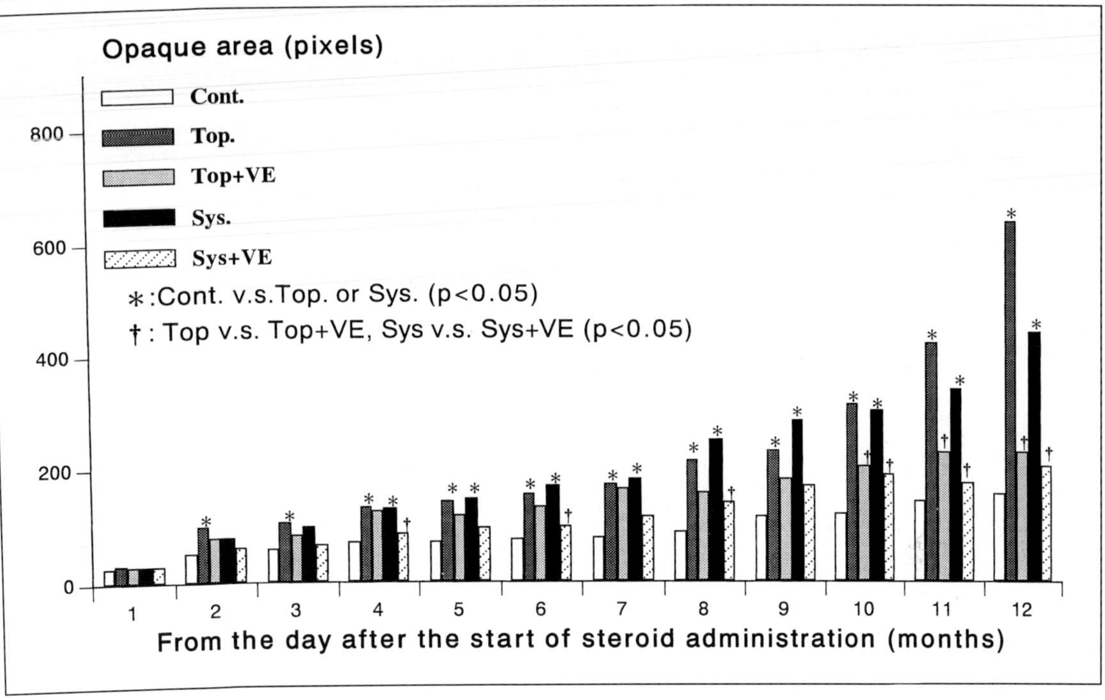

Fig. 5. Opaque area changes in the non-X-ray-irradiated left eyes during the 1-year experimental period in the 5 groups.

Discussion

Steroid-induced cataracts are well known ocular side effects in patients with long-term steroid treatment. It is impossible, however, to stop steroid therapy in patients who, for example, have undergone organ transplantation. The incidence of steroid cataract in renal transplant patients varies from 6.5 to 96% because of different follow-up duration, patients' age and methods of steroid administration [8]. However, there is no doubt that long-term steroid application is one of the risk factors of cataract formation.

The mechanisms of corticosteroid-induced cataract formation have been speculated to contain a number of factors such as inhibition of the Na,K-ATPase pump mechanism, the binding of corticosteroids to lens proteins and the subsequent formation of lysine-ketosteroid adducts, the inhibition of glucose-6-phosphate dehydrogenase, the loss of ATP, and the secondary oxidation of –SH protein groups in lysin-ketosteroid adducts leading to the aggregation of crystallins [2, 3].

In spite of numerous clinical and experimental studies, there is still no unifying concept to explain the mode of action of tocopherol [9]. VE is well known as an antioxidant. Additionally, Libondi et al. [10] reported that VE prevented changes in Na-K equilibriums and loss of protein in rat lenses incubated in lysophosphatidylcholine [10]. Cation changes and oxidative stress have been speculated to be the main factors in steroid-induced cataract formation. This is why we chose to test VE as a drug in this experiment. Furthermore, Stephens et al. [11] examined ocular VE distribution after long-term dietary depletion and supplementation, and concluded that several ocular tissues such as cornea, lens, vitreous, and sclera showed only minor changes in their levels of VE when the rats were placed on either depleted or supplemented diets [11]. These data suggest that oral VE administration would not be effective in inhibiting or delaying cataract formation in the lens.

Recently, Santen Pharmaceutical Co. Ltd. developed a VE ophthalmic solution. In our unpublished data, the VE ophthalmic solution was much better than orally administered VE. For the above reasons, we tried to apply a VE ophthalmic solution to our newly developed steroid-induced cataract rat model.

In this experiment, we found that the VE ophthalmic solution had a significant effect on steroid-induced cataract when applied both systemically and topically. The difference between the VE-treated groups (Top + VE and SYS + VE) and non-VE-treated groups (Top and Sys) was evaluated by both objective and quantitative methods. Scheimpflug image analysis enabled us to elucidate very precise lens changes [7].

Of the 2 groups receiving the VE ophthalmic solution, the efficacy of the SYS + VE group appeared earlier than that of the Top + VE group. This may be an interesting finding. In general, the steroid side effects accompanying systemic application have been thought to be more severe and of a higher incidence than those of topical steroid administration. Several cases were reviewed by Urban and Cotlier [2]. The reason for the small number of reports concerning topically administered steroid cataract is rather simple: long-term topical application of steroid is rare.

From the standpoint of lenticular toxicity of the steroid, topical administration is more dangerous than systemic administration. In fact, the lenticular concentration of prednisolone acetate in rabbits after eye drop application was much higher than that of intravenous administration [12]. This means that the lenticular steroid concentrations of the topically administered steroid groups (Top and Top + VE) might be much higher than those of the systemically administered groups (Sys and Sys + VE). Therefore, systemic administration with subsequent VE treatment (Sys + VE) was effective more quickly in the prevention of cataract progression than the Top + VE treatment (fig. 4, 5). Although the body weight fluctuations in both the VE-treated groups were a bit more extreme than those of the non VE-treated groups, the above-mentioned efficacy of VE seems to be due not to whole body improvement, but its direct efficacy for steroid-induced lenticular changes.

The precise mechanisms of the steroid-induced cataract and the efficacy of VE are still unknown. In this experiment, biochemical analysis of the rat lenses was not done. Thus, it is difficult to explain why VE prevented steroid-induced cataract. The authors, however, believe that VE is closely correlated with steroid-induced cataract. Preliminary experiments on the prevention of steroid-induced lenticular changes by a VE ophthalmic solution under a VE-deficient condition are currently in progress.

References

1 Black RL, Oglesby RB, von Sallmann I, Bunim JJ: Posterior subcapsular cataracts induced by corticosteroids in patients with rheumatoid arthritis. JAMA 1960;174:166–171.

2 Urban RC, Cotlier E: Corticosteroid-induced cataracts. Surv Ophthalmol 1986;31:102–110.

3 Harding JJ: Cataract. Biochemistry, Epidemiology and Pharmacology. London, Chapman & Hall, 1991.

4 Leske MC, Wu SH, Hyman L, Sperduto R, Underwood B, Chylack LT, Milton RC, Srivastave S, Ansari N, the Lens Opacities Case-Control Study Group: Biochemical factors in the lens opacities case-control study. Arch Ophthalmol 1995;113:1113–1119.

5 Shui YB, Kojima M, Hockwin O, Sasaki K: In vivo morphological changes in rat lenses induced by the administration of prednisolone after subliminal X-irradiation. A preliminary report. Ophthalmic Res 1995; 27:178–186.

6 Sasaki K, Sakamoto Y, Shibata T, Emori Y: The multi-purpose camera: A new anterior eye segment analysis system. Ophthalmic Res 1990;22(suppl 1):3–8.

7 Kojima M, Sasaki K: Application of a new Scheimpflug camera (EAS-1000) to animal cataract models. Ophthalmic Res 1992;24(suppl 1): 3–9.

8 Yamamura T, Takizawa A, Sasaki K: Long-term follow-up study of steroid cataracts; in Hockwin (ed): Drug-Induced Ocular Side Effects and Ocular Toxicology. Concepts Toxicol. Basel, Karger, 1987, vol 4, pp 79–86.

9 Marks J: The fat-soluble vitamins in modern medicine; in Harris RS, Munson PL, Diczfalusy E, Glover J (eds): Vitamins and Hormones: Advances in Research and Applications. New York, Academic Press, 1974, vol 32, pp 143–146.

10 Libondi T, Menzione M, Auricchio G: In vitro effects of alpha-tocopherol on lysophosphatidylcholine-induced lens damage. Exp Eye Res 1985;40:661–666.

11 Stephens RJ, Negi DS, Short SM, van Kuijk FJGM, Dratz EA, Thomas DW: Vitamin E distribution in ocular tissues following long-term dietary depletion and supplementation as determined by microdissection and gas chromatography-mass spectrometry. Exp Eye Res 1988;47: 237–245.

12 Kojima M: Drug distribution studies in single lens layers through the application of a sectioning technique; in Weisse I, Hockwin O, Green K, Tripathi RC (eds): Ocular Toxicology. New York, Plenum Press, 1995, pp 121–134.

Ophthalmic Research

Ophthalmic Res 1996;28(suppl 2):72–77

Kazuko Kitagawa[a]
Yasuo Sakamoto[a]
Kazuyuki Sasaki[a]
Hirohiko Hanaki[b]

[a] Department of Ophthalmology, Kanazawa Medical University, Uchinada, Ishikawa, and
[b] Nidek Co. Ltd., Gamagoori, Aichi, Japan

Evaluation of Transparency and Barrier Function of the Cornea by Scheimpflug Images

Key Words
Scheimpflug imaging
Anterior eye segment analysis system
Fluorescein sodium
Light scattering
Tear fluid dynamics
Dry eye
Keratitis

Abstract
Two new methods of corneal analysis with Scheimpflug images will be introduced in this paper. The first study was to document the light scattering of the cornea itself using a newly modified Scheimpflug camera with higher magnification. Details of the slit images of the cornea could be evaluated more precisely than those of images taken with an existing camera. The second study was to evaluate the corneal epithelial barrier function by measuring the intensity of the light scattering originating from instilled fluorescein excited through filters. Fluorescein accumulation in the damaged epithelium and diffusion with time into the stromal tissue could be observed in two-dimensional images and the changes could also be documented by measuring the intensity and extent of light scattering. These newly developed methods will be useful for studies of the cornea.

Introduction

Scheimpflug photography was initially aimed at the analysis of morphological or transparency changes in the lens. However, the analysis of Scheimpflug images has opened up the possibility of its wide application to other parts of the anterior eye segment, as the authors have demonstrated with tear-fluid dynamics [1] and hard contact lens fitting [2]. Since it has not been applied to investigations of corneal or tear-fluid changes until quite recently, further studies are necessary before it can be established.

In the studies cited above it was discovered that the images of the cornea, including pre-

KARGER

E-Mail karger@karger.ch
Fax + 41 61 306 12 34
http://www.karger.ch

© 1996 S. Karger AG, Basel
0030–3747/96/0288–0072$10.00/0

Kazuko Kitagawa, MD
Department of Ophthalmology
Kanazawa Medical University
Uchinada, Ishikawa 920-02 (Japan)

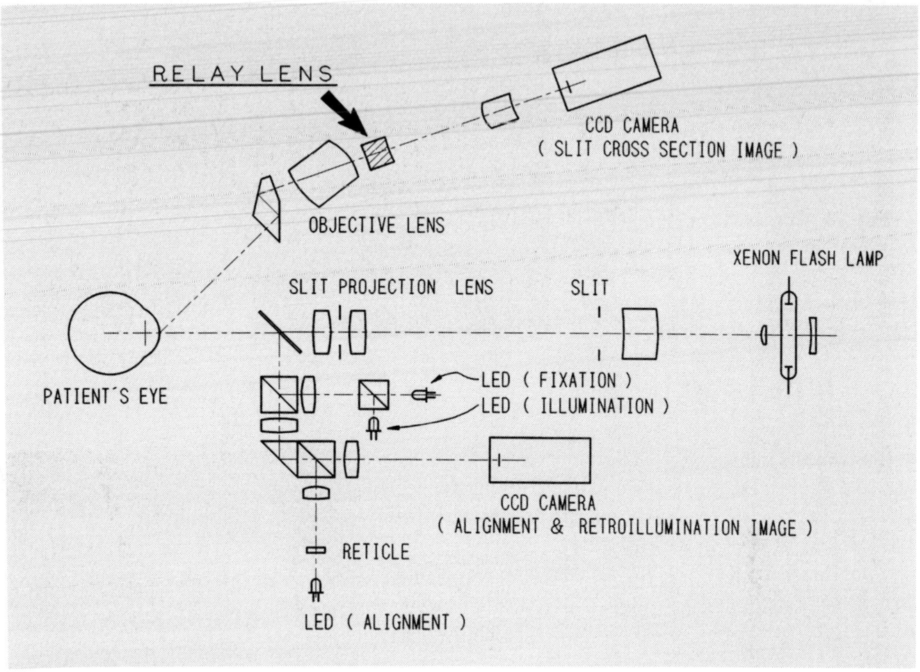

Fig. 1. Diagram of the system with high magnification. Arrow: an inserted relay lens. LED: Light-emitting diode.

corneal tear film obtained with the EAS–1000 [1], were too small for precise analysis and that the optical system of the Scheimpflug camera needed to be modified for higher magnification. Therefore, the images of several cases with corneal disease were analyzed using an original EAS–1000 system and a modified camera. The transparency and barrier function of the cornea were evaluated using these systems in this paper.

Subjects and Methods

20 volunteers with normal corneas and 4 patients with corneal diseases were selected for studies to evaluate corneal transparency (ages 13–82 years). Fifteen patients with corneal epithelial lesions were selected to study the corneal epithelial barrier function (ages 23–80 years), including 12 cases of Sjögren's syndrome, 1 case with suspected corneal spheroidal degeneration, 1 case of recurrent erosion, and 1 case of bacterial corneal ulcer.

The Scheimpflug camera techniques applied were the original anterior eye segment analysis equipment (EAS–1000, Nidek) and a newly modified camera. The system of the modified camera is principally the same as that of the original, except for a relay lens which was inserted in front of the CCD camera (fig. 1). The magnification of an image taken with the modified camera was 6.25 times higher than that of the original camera (fig. 2). To test the corneal epithelial barrier function, 1 µl of a 1% fluorescein sodium solution was instilled into the cul-de-sac of the patients as an indicator of light emitted in the target regions. In order to detect the fluorescence of fluorescein sodium, an excitation interference filter of 465–520 nm and a Wratten No. 15 barrier filter were applied to the EAS-1000. The observation of the patients with fluorescein sodium solution lasted from 15 s to 15 min. Light-scattering intensity at the target region was expressed as a CCD count detected by linear densitometry (equipped in the software of the original image-analysis device). Corneal epithelial damage was evaluated by measuring the

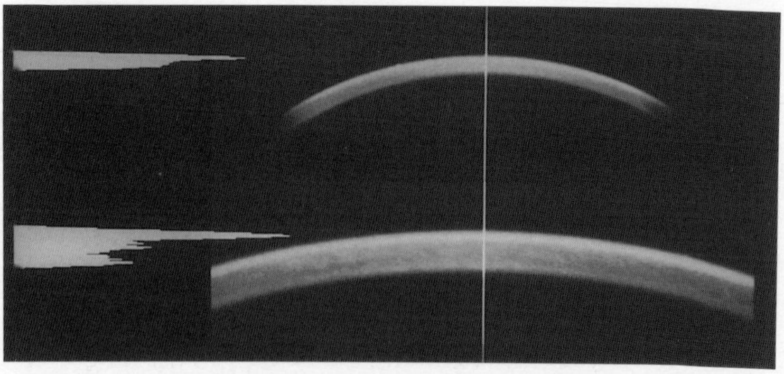

Fig. 2. Comparison of a conventional image (top) and a magnified image (bottom). Linear densitometries at the optical axis of each image are shown on the left.

intensity of the light scattering that originated from the retained fluorescein at the level of the corneal surface after instillation and by evaluating the degree of diffusion into the stromal tissue with time.

The transparencies of the normal and opacified corneas were objectively evaluated through light-scattering intensities at a focused location using a modified camera.

Results

Evaluation of Corneal Transparency

Light-scattering intensity patterns taken with the EAS-1000 and the modified camera were principally the same (fig. 2). The magnified images showed more detailed information on the whole layers of the cornea. The pattern is mainly constituted by the initial rise at the surface followed by gradually decreasing light with small fluctuations corresponding to the corneal stromal tissue, and a lower peak at the deepest layer of the cornea. In magnified images of the transparent corneas of normal volunteers, light-scattering intensities of the first and the last rise were measured at the optical axis. They ranged from 110 to 126 and from 70 to 92 CCT, respectively, and had a tendency to increase with age. The expanded affected stromal regions of the 4 diseased corneas were precisely detectable by the magnified images (fig. 3).

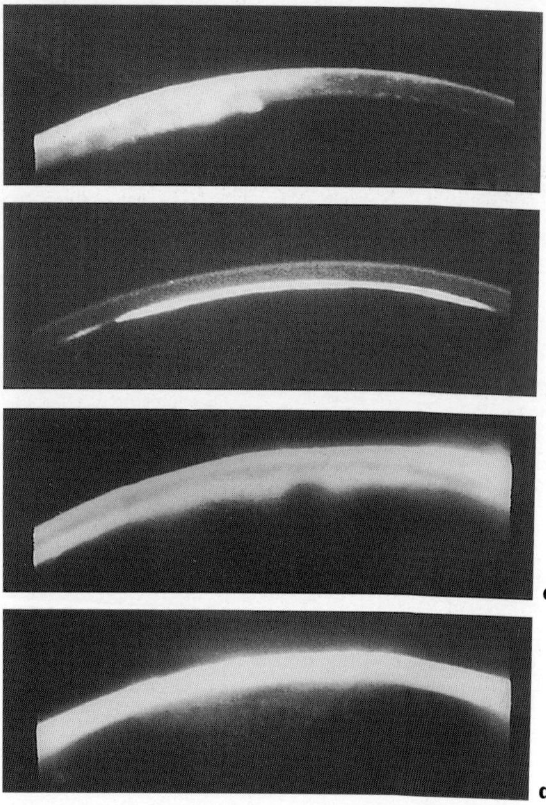

a

b

c

d

Fig. 3. The scattering pattern of magnified images of the cornea with various diseases. The distribution of the lesion can be observed more precisely. The degrees of opacity are measurable quantitatively using densitometrical analysis. **a** Corneal edema due to herpes zoster keratitis. **b** Internal corneal scar due to keratomycosis. **c** Corneal edema due to absolute glaucoma. **d** Corneal opacity of Schnyder's corneal dystrophy.

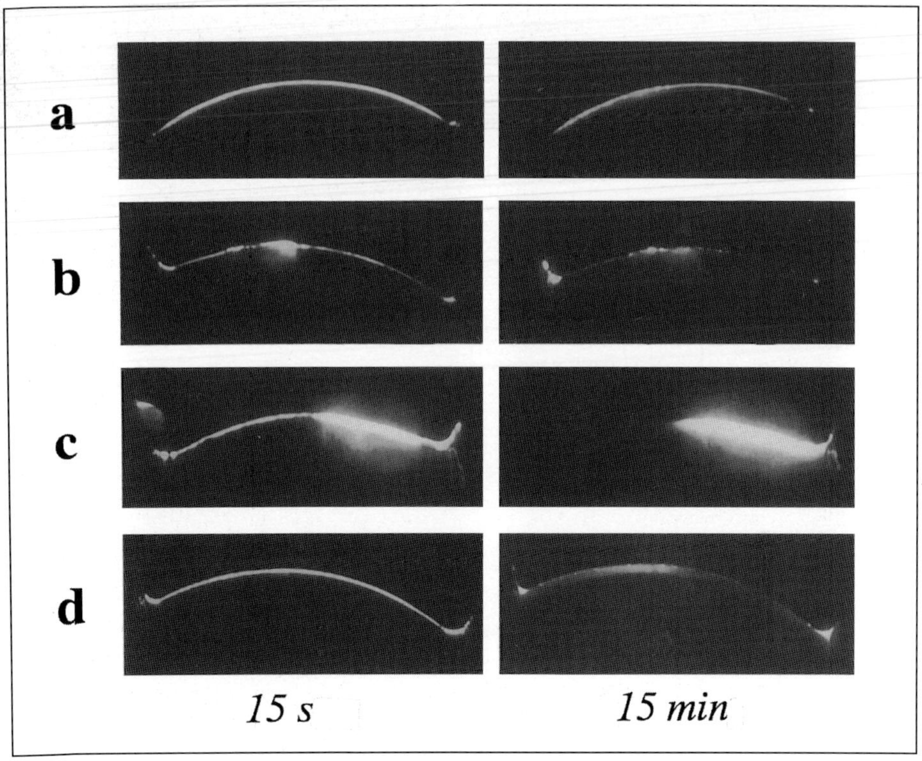

Fig. 4. The patterns of fluorescein diffusion into the cornea with various conditions 15 s and 15 min after instillation. In 3 cases, except for a case of Sjögren's syndrome (**a**), excretion of fluorescein from the precorneal tear fluid was normal. **a** Corneal epithelial lesion caused by Sjögren's syndrome. Fluorescein was retained in the tear fluid and accumulated at the ocular surface. Diffusion was observed only in the superficial layer of the cornea. **b** Corneal epithelial degeneration, suspected spheroidal degeneration. Fluorescein was localized only on the surface of the lesion. **c** Bacterial corneal ulcer. Remarkable staining and the diffusion of fluorescein into the anterior chamber was observed at the damage site. In the other portion of the cornea, no light scattering was detectable. The damage to barrier function was thought to be almost normal except for the ulcerative area. **d** Recurrent corneal erosion. In this case, epithelial healing was achieved except for superficial punctate keratopathy, but fluorescein diffused and stained all layers of the cornea from the site of the lesion.

Evaluation or Corneal Epithelial Barrier Function

Corneal barrier function was evaluated through the fluorescence diffusion mode. The light-scattering intensity originating from fluorescein sodium diffusion into the stromal tissues of eyes with normal corneas was under the level of intensity measurable [1]. In the eyes with corneal epithelial damage, the diffusion of fluorescein was observed from the affected corneal surface into the stromal tissue with time. When epithelial damage was severe, fluorescein was also observed in the aqueous fluid of the anterior chamber. The mode of diffusion, speed of fluorescein penetration toward the anterior chamber or expansion of the diffusion area varied according to the type and severity of the disease (fig. 4). In

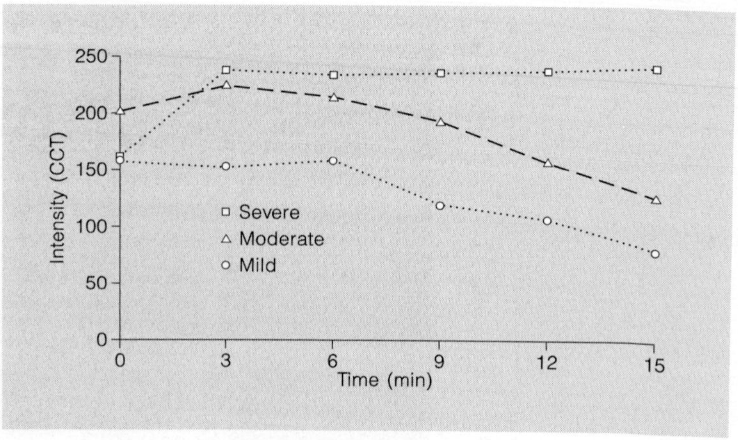

Fig. 5. Light-scattering-changes with time at the optical axis in Sjögren's syndrome after instillation of fluorescein. Three typical cases are demonstrated.

the eyes with Sjögren's syndrome, the fluorescein concentration in the tear fluid decreased more slowly than in normal eyes and accumulated in the damaged epithelium (fig. 4a, 5).

Discussion

The application of Scheimpflug photography to the clinical field was initiated by Niesel [3] and Brown [4] at the end of the 1960s using their own handmade cameras. Since the late 1970s, several types of Scheimpflug cameras have been developed and become commercially available. Although the field of application has been limited mainly to the lens, several other applications of this photography have been proposed. Among these, research in to the corneal field and tear dynamics is in progress [1, 2]. Although images taken by conventional slit lamp photography were also applied, the analysis of documented changes was subjective. Application of the Scheimpflug camera has now made objective analysis of findings with two-dimensional images possible [1, 5], and that of three-dimensional images will be possible in the near future. This has already been established in principle for the lens [6].

Detection of fluorescein originating from an instilled fluorescein sodium solution through a Scheimpflug camera will make possible the analysis of precorneal tear film dynamics and the barrier function of the corneal epithelium by densitometrical analysis of Scheimpflug images. The intensity at the ocular surface returned to baseline in 6 min in young subjects and in 15 min in older subjects [1]. As shown in this paper, the retention of fluorescein is quite abnormal. Morphological analysis of these patients will be informative in evaluating the extent of damage to the corneal epithelial barrier function.

In patients with Sjögren's syndrome, the fluorescein concentration in precorneal tear fluid remained at a high level for a longer period. To make the contact time with the dye uniform, techniques such as washing the dye out of the cul-de-sac will be needed in order to compare the epithelial barrier functions of various corneal diseases. Nevertheless, the analysis shown here makes it possible to observe the natural course of the dynamics of instilled fluorescein in each patient.

Magnified images are more informative for the study of the cornea, and several experiments including fluorescein dynamics through the use of this equipment are expected. We believe that the morphological techniques shown in this study will also be useful for both clinical and basic studies of the cornea. Modern surgical techniques for the cornea performed by an excimer laser need precise observation and morphological analysis of the treated cornea. Scheimpflug photography may also be a useful tool for this purpose, and the magnified images shown in this study would be ideal. Further examination utilizing the modified camera is in progress, including the development of a Scheimpflug camera for corneal use.

References

1 Kitagawa K, Sasaki K, Sakamoto Y: Application of Scheimpflug photography to the study of tear fluid dynamics. Ophthalmic Res 1994;26 (suppl 1):39.

2 Kitagawa K, Sakamoto Y, Sasaki K: Observation of hard contact lens-wearing eyes using a Scheimpflug camera (in Japanese). J Jpn CL Soc 1993;35:273.

3 Niesel P: Spaltlampen Photographie mit der Haag-Streit Spaltlampe 900. Ophthalmologica 1966;151:489.

4 Brown N: Slit-image photography. Trans Ophthal Soc UK 1969;89: 398.

5 Busin M, Spitznas M, Hockwin O: Evaluation of functional and morphologic parameters of the cornea after epikeratophakia using prelathed, lyophilized tissue. Ophthalmology 1990;97:330.

6 Sakamoto Y, Sasaki K: Computed tomographic images and three dimentional expression of crystalline lens findings from multiple slices of Scheimpflug slit images. Ophthalmic Res 1995;27(suppl):94.

Ophthalmic Research

Ophthalmic Res 1996;28(suppl 2):78–85

Gijs F.J.M. Vrensen
Anneke de Wolf

Department of Morphology, The Netherlands Ophthalmic Research Institute, Amsterdam, The Netherlands

Calcium Distribution in the Human Eye Lens

Key Words
Lens
Human
Calcium
Ultrastructure
Cytochemistry

Abstract
The distribution of calcium in the human eye lens was investigated using the oxalate-pyroantimonate technique. In epithelial cells and superficial cortical fibers calcium is sequestered and tightly bound to proteins in the endoplasmic reticulum, nuclear envelope, Golgi cisterns and mitochondria. In intermediate fibers these cell organelles are broken down and the liberated calcium is ionically bound to the phospholipids at the extracellular side of the fiber-limiting membrane. It is argued that calcium is probably additionally bound to β-crystallin. This site-specific variation in calcium storage might explain the deeper cortical localization of early focal dot opacities and retrodots.

Introduction

In a recent review paper Duncan et al. [1] discussed the strategic role of calcium homeostasis in maintaining lens transparency. On account of observations that freely exchangeable calcium forms only a very minor fraction of the total lens calcium it can be concluded that the majority of calcium must be somehow cytoplasmically sequestered in the epithelial cells and lens fibers. Since upon ageing the calcium content of the lens considerably increases without leading to an increase in visible opacities [2] the sequestration capacity must be in excess and able to accommodate additional amounts of calcium entering the lens. Mitochondria are able to take up large amounts of calcium and serve as calcium sinks. The endoplasmic reticulum including the nuclear envelope is more efficient in regulating the amount of free vs. bound calcium [3]. Regarding the calcium sequestering organelles it has to be realized that upon maturation there is a complete breakdown of the

KARGER
E-Mail karger@karger.ch
Fax + 41 61 306 12 34
http://www.karger.ch

© 1996 S. Karger AG, Basel
0030–3747/96/0288–0078$10.00/0

Dr. Gijs F.J.M. Vrensen
Department of Morphology
The Netherlands Ophthalmic Research Institute
PO Box 12141
NL–1100 AC Amsterdam (The Netherlands)

nuclei, cisterns of the endoplasmic reticulum and mitochondria [4]. Since the fiber cells do not render opaque we must assume that the large amounts of calcium liberated during this breakdown of the stores are accommodated by other cytoplasmic stores. In a recent cytochemical study by Vrensen et al. [5] it was shown that in rat lenses the limiting membranes of lens fibers are able to bind considerable amounts of calcium. The present cytochemical investigation aimed to study this shift in calcium binding in clear human donor lenses.

Materials and Methods

Eight clear human eye lenses, varying in age between 19 and 85 years were obtained from the Cornea Bank Amsterdam (Head: Dr. *E. Pels*). Time between enucleation and lens extraction was maximally 16 h. After extraction they were immediately fixed according to the oxalate-pyroantimonate technique as described by Van Reempts et al. [6]. After embedding in epoxy resin ultrathin sections were cut, stained with uranyl acetate and lead citrate and inspected in a Philips CM12 transmission electron microscope (Philips Industries, Eindhoven, The Netherlands).

Results

Although some small differences in the amount of calcium precipitates were found, depending on donor age and time between death and extraction, the observations were very consistent among lenses. As outlined previously [5, 7] the calcium precipitates comprise calcium antimonate which replaces the original calcium oxalate during the postfixation procedure. In addition, the calcium precipitates only reflect the presence of 'loosely', ionically, bound calcium; free calcium is washed out and calcium tightly bound to proteins is not free to complex with the oxalate.

As illustrated in survey pictures of the equatorial cortex (fig. 1) calcium precipitates are almost absent in the epithelium and the first 5–10 cortical fibers. In the deeper cortex an abundancy of calcium precipitates is observed. At higher magnifications (fig. 2) it could be shown that epithelial cells and first cortical fibers have a few calcium precipitates in mitochondria, Golgi fields and elements of the endoplasmic reticulum. In the deeper, 'intermediate' cortex (fig. 3) calcium precipitates are abundant in the nuclear envelope, the endoplasmic reticulum and the mitochondria. Moreover, some fibers (fig. 1, 3a) exhibit numerous precipitates in the cytoplasm and along the fiber-limiting membranes. The membrane precipitates are all along the fiber surface but are absent at the gap junctions (fig. 4). Progressing to the deeper cortex, beyond the zone of nuclear breakdown, precipitates along the membranes remain present but finally nearly disappear in the perinuclear cortex and nucleus (fig. 5). In the anterior and posterior regions a similar calcium precipitate gradient is observed with the restriction that the amount of precipitate is less pronounced.

Discussion

The distribution of calcium precipitates in the human eye lens, reflecting the distribution of 'loosely' or ionically bound calcium [5, 7], is essentially the same as in the rat lens [5]: few precipitates in the epithelial cells and superficial fibers, appearance of abundant precipitates along the fiber-limiting membranes in the deeper cortex and gradual disappearance towards the perinuclear cortex and nucleus. In several respects the observations in human lenses deviate from those in young (10- to 12-week-old) rat lenses: (i) The zone of precipitate-free superficial fibers is much smaller in human lenses. Upon aging there is

1

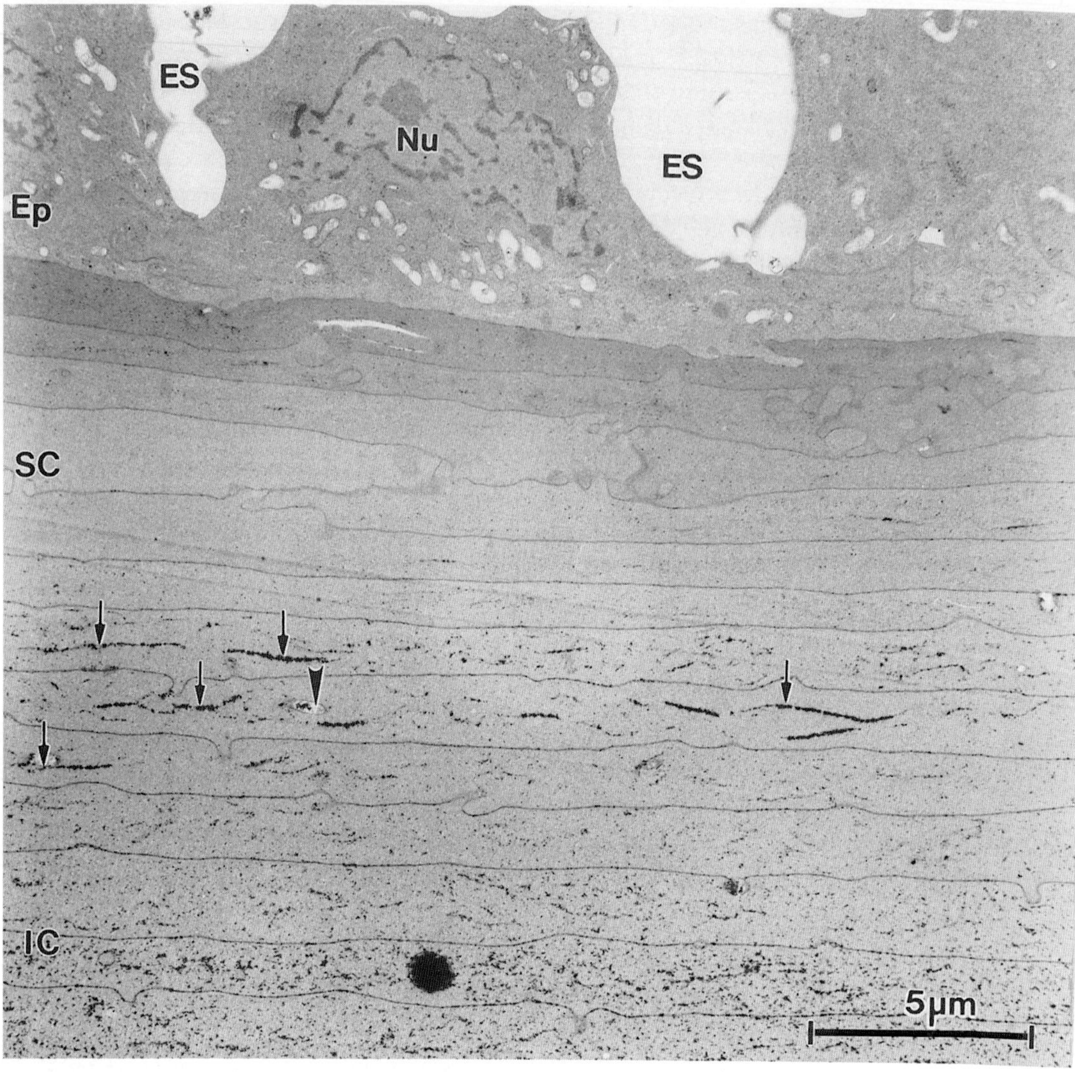

Fig. 1. Example of survey picture in the equatorial region of a human lens illustrating the paucity of calcium precipitates in the epithelium (EP) and superficial cortex (SC). Somewhat deeper lens fibers are characterized by abundant precipitates in mitochondria (arrowhead) and endoplasmic reticulum (arrows). In the intermediate cortex (IC) precipitates are found scattered throughout the fiber cytoplasm. Nu = Nucleus; ES = extracellular space commonly observed in human donor lenses.

Fig. 2. Medium-power micrographs illustrating the presence of calcium precipitates in the cisterns of the Golgi fields (GF) and mitochondria (M) of epithelial cells (**a**). In superficial fibers (**b**) precipitates are found in mitochondria (M) and associated with cisterns of the endoplasmic reticulum (ER). Nu = Nucleus.

Fig. 3. In intermediate fibers calcium precipitates are found scattered throughout the cytoplasm and localized in or close to the mitochondria (M) and endoplasmic reticulum (ER). As illustrated in **b**, the nuclear envelope is partly filled with precipitates (arrows). Nu = Nucleus.

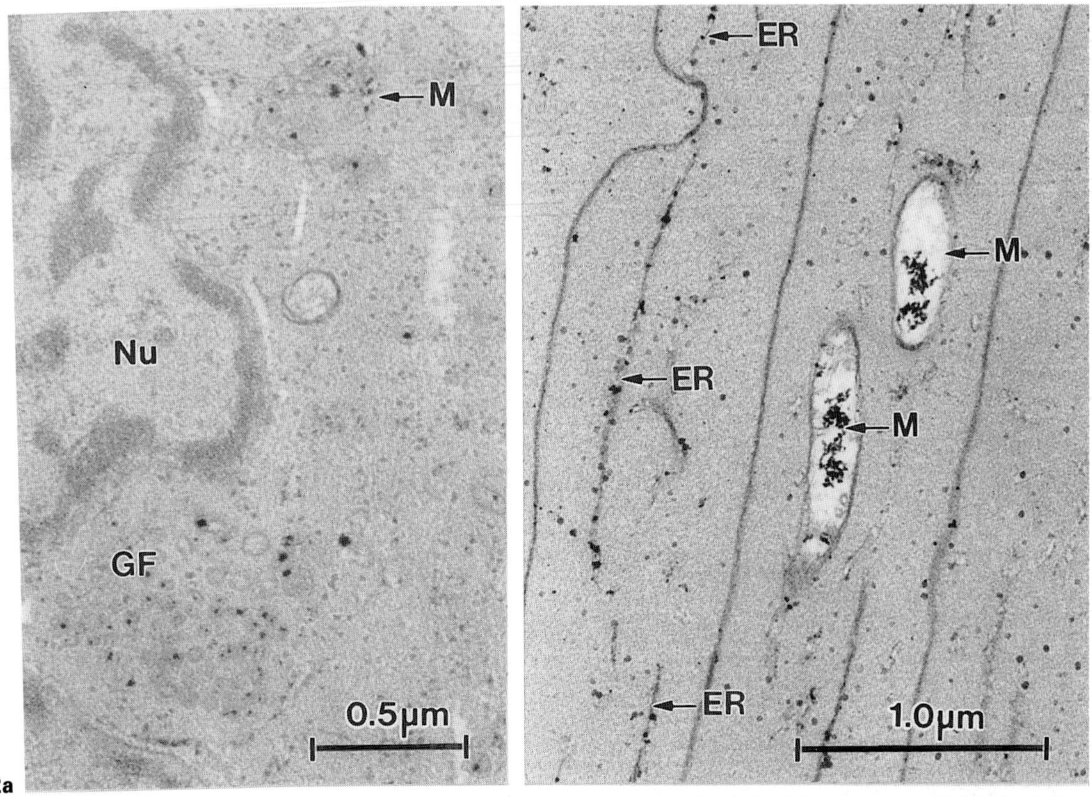

2a

2b

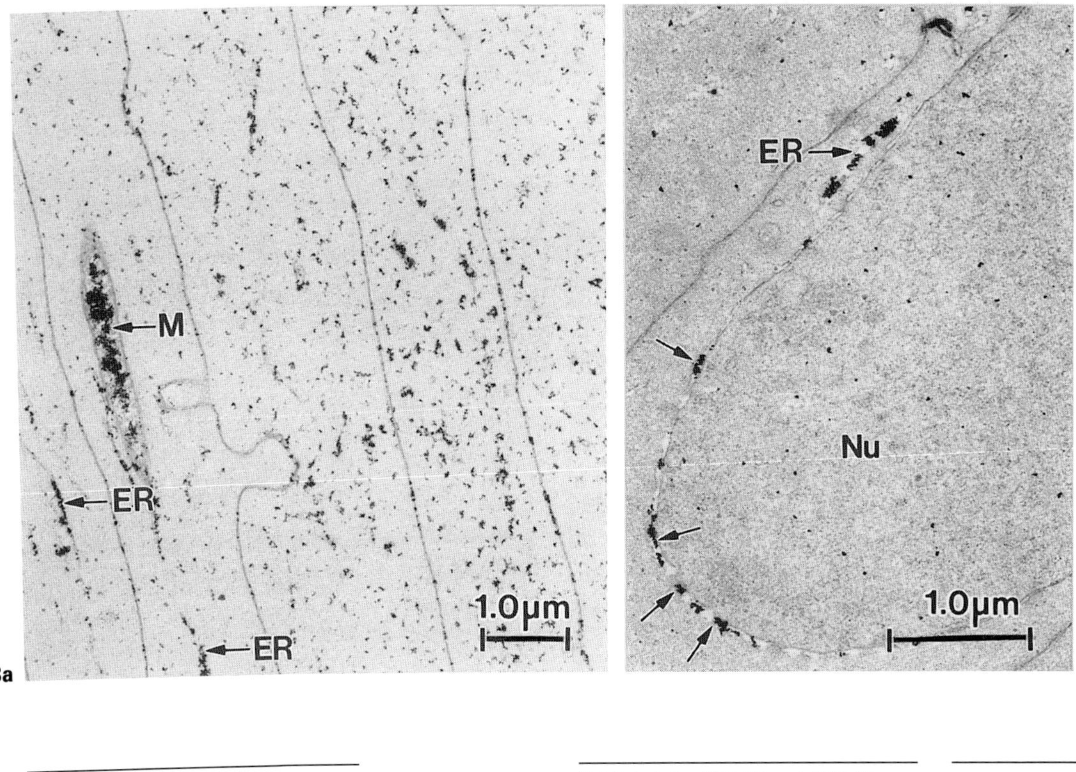

3a

3b

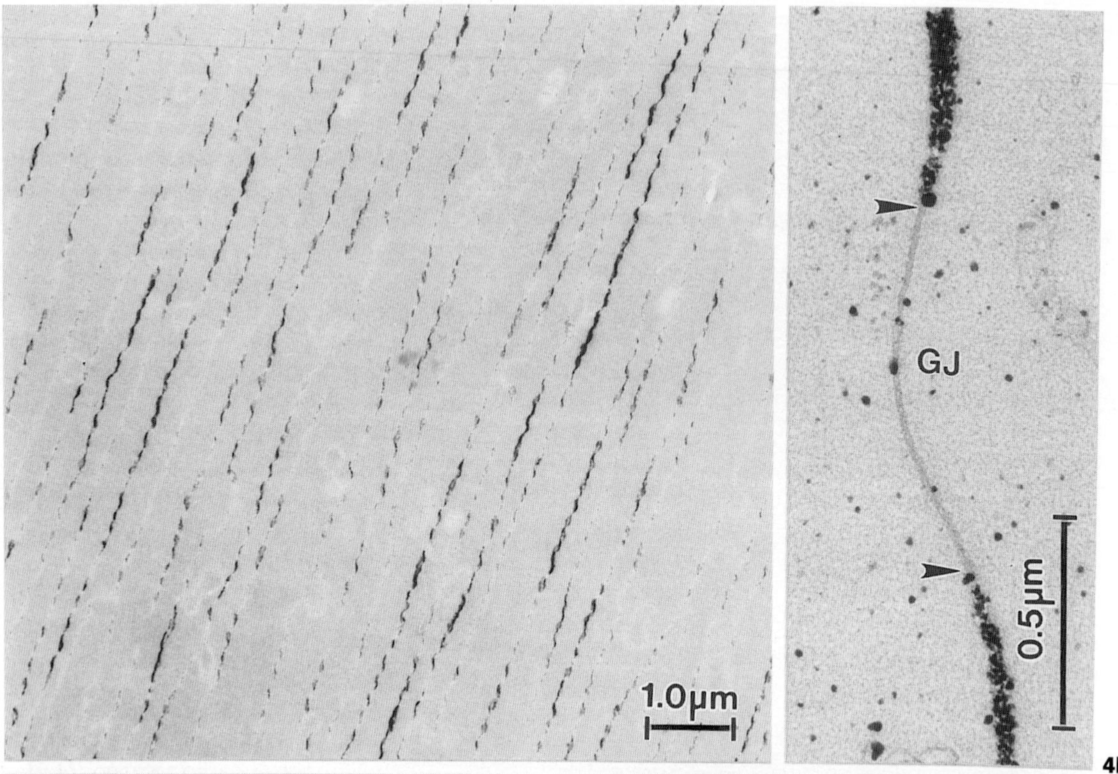

4a 4b

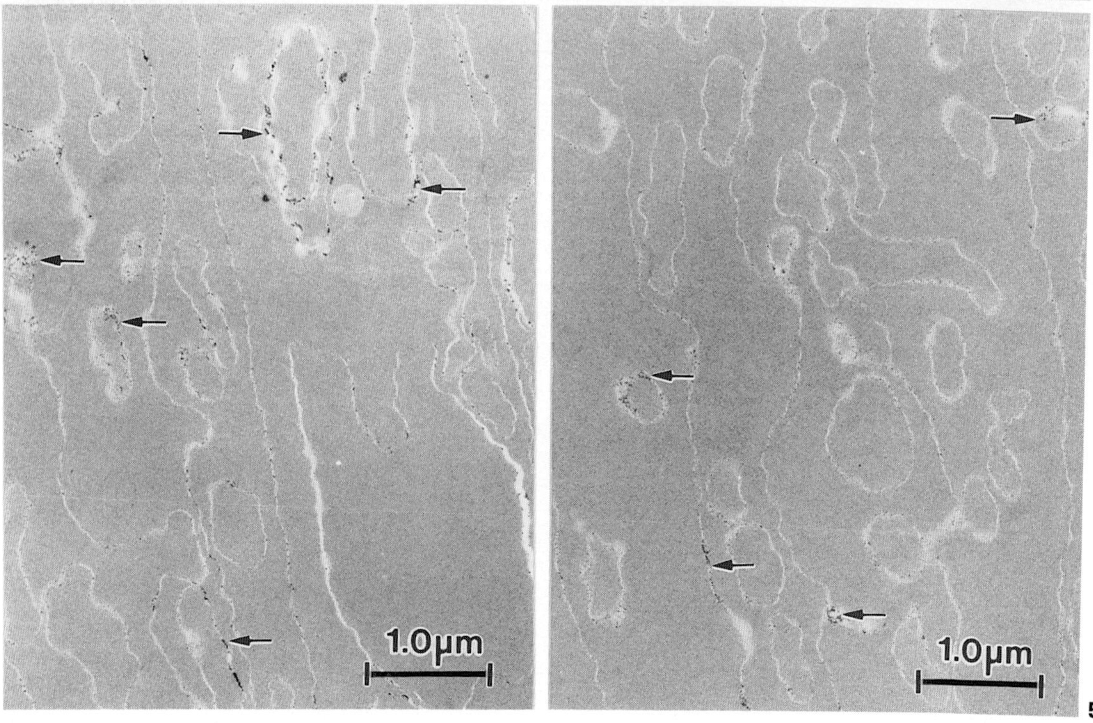

5a 5b

a slowdown of mitotic activity in the germinative layer and therefore the zone of differentiating and maturing fibers must be smaller. Since as detailed below, maturation is accompanied by the breakdown of calcium-sequestering organelles, thus setting free the sequestered calcium, this smaller precipitate-free zone in humans is not surprising. (ii) In rat lenses no precipitates were found in the cytoplasm, the endoplasmic reticulum, the nuclear envelope and the mitochondria of untreated control lenses. Their presence in the human lenses may be due to postmortem effects and therefore be artefactual. In recent experiments [Sanderson et al., pers. commun.] dimethyl sulfoxide (DMSO) was used to enhance the penetration into the lens fibers of calpain inhibitors. In these DMSO-treated lenses precipitates were found in the cytoplasm, the endoplasmic reticulum, the nuclear envelope and the mitochondria of intermediate cortical fibers. DMSO is known to 'weaken' the calcium-binding properties of proteins thus making this calcium available for trapping by oxalate. This means that in these DMSO-treated rat lenses, and probably also in the human postmortem lenses, the precipitates in the fiber cytoplasm and organelles most likely reflect protein-bound calcium.

This accidental DMSO and postmortem effect on bound lens calcium and the regular localization of ionically bound calcium allows us to give a comprehensive description of calcium localization in the eye lens. In the epithelial cells and the metabolically active superficial fibers the far majority (>99.0% [1]) of calcium is sequestered and tightly bound in the endoplasmic reticulum (calsequestrin), nuclear envelope, Golgi cisterns and mitochondria. This calcium can be mobilized by the cellular mechanisms as for instance described by Duncan et al. [1]. Upon final maturation of the lens fibers the fiber cell organelles are broken down. This process is accompanied by a 'weakening' of the tightly bound sequestered calcium and emptying of the stores. This calcium is then temporarily readily accessible for trapping by the oxalate and is found as precipitates in the cytoplasm and along the fiber-limiting membranes. This is in line with the electrophysiological observation by Duncan and Jacob [8] that the highest concentration of free calcium is in the intermediate cortex. The precipitates along the fiber-limiting membranes are most likely due to binding of calcium to negatively charged phospholipids [5]. Recently, Van Marle et al. [9] have further analyzed this, using electron-microscopic tomography, and they concluded that the calcium is exclusively bound to the extracellular side of the membranes. The paucity of precipitates along the fiber-limiting membranes in the deep cortex and nucleus may partly be the consequence of the decrease in charged phospholipids and the increase in uncharged cholesterol during maturation of lens fibers [10–12]. Furthermore, it cannot be ruled out that insufficient diffusion of the oxalate into these deeper lens regions plays a role in this. However, the total calcium content of the intermediate and deep cortex is not much lower if at all than of the superficial cortex. This leaves us to explain the tight binding of calcium in these deeper zones. In a series of studies Sharma and Balasubramanian [13] have shown that β-crystallin has calcium-binding properties and additionally is present in large amounts in lens fibers. Although β-crystallin has low-affinity calcium binding the temporary abundancy of free calcium in the

Fig. 4. Beyond the intermediate zone calcium is mainly found along the fiber-limiting membranes. At high magnification the gap junctions (GJ) proved to be largely free of precipitate.

Fig. 5. In deep cortical (**a**), perinuclear (**b**) and nuclear fibers, the amount of calcium precipitates (arrows) is gradually decreasing.

intermediate zone, due to the breakdown of cellular calcium stores, favors the β-crystallin binding of calcium. The observed calcium-induced conformational changes in β-crystallin [13] may further stabilize this calcium binding especially under the low ionic strength conditions in the lens.

The possible consequences of these local variations in specific calcium storage sites are not yet understood. It is beyond doubt that the homeostasis of calcium plays an important role in lens transparency and that in many cases cataract is associated with increased calcium levels. It is also commonly noticed that clear and light-scattering areas are juxtapositioned, suggesting uncoupling between neighboring groups of lens fibers. It has also been shown that early focal opacifications are located in the intermediate cortex [14] indicating that the intermediate lens fibers are most vulnerable to cataractous risk factors. This may not be surprising in view of the transition of organelle-sequestered calcium to phospholipid and β-crystallin-bound calcium in this region. Another example of the vulnerability of the transitional intermediate zone has been given by Vrensen et al. [15]. Retrodots, i.e. round-to-oval birefringent bodies (80–500 μm), are mainly located in this zone. As measured by X-ray microanalysis the majority proved to consist of accumulation of calcium phosphate crystals. Detailed ultrastructural analysis further showed that they are associated with local disturbances of the membranes, possibly induced by oxidative stress. Membrane ruptures certainly will give rise to liberation of calcium which in turn will lead to breakdown of phospholipids due to the protein kinase C-induced enhancement of phospholipase activity. The phosphorus resulting from the phospholipid breakdown will trap the available calcium and therefore will stop the process. The large amounts of membrane-bound calcium explains the extensiveness and large size of the crystals. Despite these examples it will be evident that further detailed studies are needed before the relation between the site-specific calcium stores and cataractous changes are fully appreciated.

Acknowledgements

The authors are indebted to the co-workers of the Cornea Bank Amsterdam (Head: Dr. *E. Pels*) for providing the human donor lenses. We thank the Foundation BIS (Leiden) for collecting the donor lenses. The secretarial assistance of Mrs. R. Grimbergen-Wiersma and the photographic assistance of Mr. N. Bakker and Mr. T. Put are acknowledged. The critical discussions with Drs. J. van Marle and Y. Sharma have importantly contributed to this paper. This work is carried out within the framework of the European Concerted Action on 'The role of membranes in lens ageing and cataract' (BMH1-CT93-1650).

References

1 Duncan G, Williams MR, Riach RA: Calcium, cell signalling and cataract. Prog Ret Eye Res 1994;13:623–652.

2 Duncan G, Hightower KR, Gandolfi SA, Tomlinson J, Maraini G: Human lens membrane cation permeability increases with age. Invest Ophthalmol Vis Sci 1989;30:1855–1859.

3 Godfrand T: Pharmacology of calcium antagonists; in Marmé D (ed): Calcium and Cell Physiology. Heidelberg, Springer, 1985, pp 204–226.

4 Bassnett S: The fate of the Golgi apparatus and the endoplasmic reticulum during lens fiber cell differentiation. Invest Ophthalmol Vis Sci 1995;36:1793–1803.

5 Vrensen G, Sanderson J, Willekens B, Duncan G: Calcium localization and ultrastructure of clear and pCMPS treated rat lenses. Invest Ophthalmol Vis Sci 1995;36:2287–2295.

6 Van Reempts J, Borgers M, Offner F: Ultrastructural localization of calcium in the rat retina with a combined oxalate-pyroantimonate technique. Histochem J 1982;14:517–522.

7 Mentré P, Halpern S: Localization of cations by pyroantimonate. II. Electron probe microanalysis of calcium and sodium in skeletal muscle of mouse. J Histochem Cytochem 1988;36:55–64.
8 Duncan G, Jacob T: Calcium and the physiology of cataract; in Nugent J, Whelan J (eds): Human Cataract Formation. Ciba Found Symp 1988; 106:132–148.
9 Van Marle J, Vrensen G, Jonges R, De Wolf A, Van Veen H: Interfibre calcium precipitates are restricted to the intercellular phase: an electron microscopic tomographic study. Vision Res 1995;35S:73.
10 Li L-K, So L, Spector A: Membrane cholesterol and phospholipid in consecutive concentric sections of human lenses. J Lipid Res 1985;26: 600–609.
11 Duindam J, Vrensen GFJM, Otto C, Puppels GJ, Greve J: New approach to assess the cholesterol distribution in the eye lens: Confocal Raman microspectroscopy and filipin probing. J Lipid Res 1995;36:1139–1145.
12 Duindam J, Vrensen GFJM, Otto C, Greve J: Aging affects the conformation of cholesterol in the human eye lens. Ophthalmic Res 1996;28(suppl 1):86–91.
13 Sharma Y, Balasubramanian D: Calcium binding properties of beta-crystallins. Ophthalmic Res 1996; 28(suppl 1):44–47.
14 Vrensen G, Willekens B: Classification and prevalence of early senile lens opacities in human donor eyes; in Hockwin O, Sasaki K, Leske MC (eds): Risk Factors for Cataract Development. Dev Ophthalmol. Basel, Karger, 1989, vol 17, pp 181–187.
15 Vrensen GFJM, Willekens B, De Jong PTVM, Shun-Shin GA, Brown NP, Bron AJ: Heterogeneity in ultrastructure and elemental composition of perinuclear lens retrodots. Invest Ophthalmol Vis Sci 1994;35: 199–206.

Ophthalmic Research

Ophthalmic Res 1996;28(suppl 2):86–91

A. Wegener
H. Laser

Department of Experimental Ophthalmology, Rheinische Friedrich-Wilhelms University, Bonn, Germany

Imaging of the Spatial Density Distribution on the Capsule of the Lens with Scheimpflug Photography

Key Words
Scheimpflug imaging
Human lens
Capsular density
Geometric correction

Abstract
The density characteristics of the anterior and posterior surfaces of the lens, although of primary importance for its optical quality, are difficult to determine. Scheimpflug photography, however, allows distinct density measurements from the optical axis towards the periphery with the only limitation of a sufficient mydriasis, so that a 3-dimensional scatter profile of both capsular surfaces can be calculated via multilinear densitometric evaluation of a sufficient number of meridians. On this methodical basis, we analysed Scheimpflug images recorded with the Topcon SL-45 on Kodak T-Max 400 film from 25 patients in an age range between 19 and 63 years. Images from the 0° + 45° meridians were scanned with multilinear microdensitometry and the data computed to get a density profile. In general, most scattering profiles show a marked interindividual variability. Nevertheless, a general trend can be established between the periphery and the center of the anterior and posterior capsules: (a) the anterior capsule generally has a higher density than the posterior; (b) in most cases, the center of the posterior capsule has a higher density than the periphery; (c) the anterior capsule has a more uniform spatial density distribution in all cases. From the cases evaluated, it can be concluded that the density of the peripheral posterior capsule is more importantly influenced by shading effects of the iris, so that geometrical correction is needed.

Introduction

The spatial distribution of light scattering in the eye lens, thus its density profile, is of primary importance not only for the optical imaging quality of the lens in normal subjects, but even more so in cataract patients. For the visual function of the patient, especially the density profiles of the anterior and posterior capsules (= borderlines with a change in refractive index) are of importance, as they optically influence the focus of the image more than the deeper cortex and the nucleus.

Among the optical techniques that allow monitoring of the anterior eye segment, Scheimpflug photography is the only method which allows exact and reproducible recording and evaluation of density profiles from the optical axis of the lens to the periphery, including both capsules [1–4]. The limitation for documentation of the posterior capsule, however, is the degree of mydriasis that can be induced.

KARGER

E-Mail karger@karger.ch
Fax + 41 61 306 12 34
http://www.karger.ch

© 1996 S. Karger AG, Basel
0030–3747/96/0288–0086$10.00/0

Dr. Alfred Wegener
Department of Experimental Ophthalmology
Rheinische Friedrich-Wilhelms University
Sigmund-Freud-Strasse 25
D–53105 Bonn (Germany)

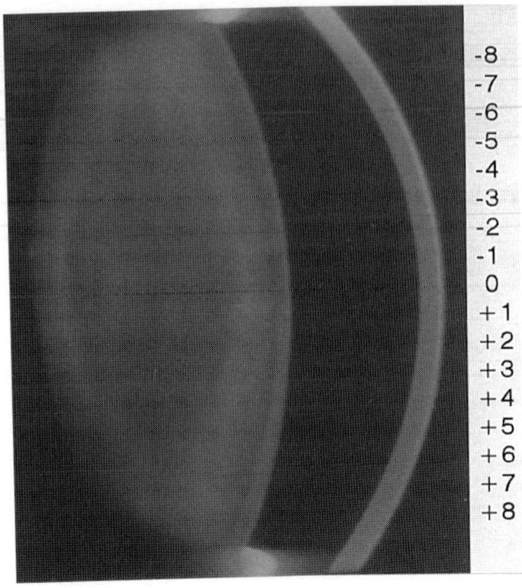

Fig. 1. Scheimpflug image of a normal human cornea and lens with the plains of parallel multilinear microdensitometric evaluation.

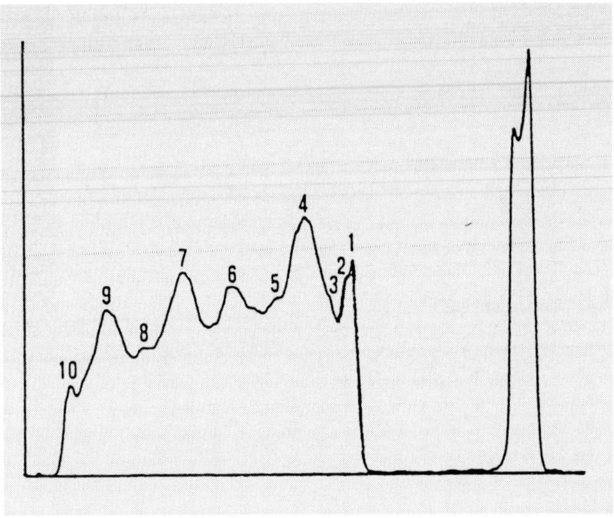

Fig. 2. Densitometric scan showing the corneal peak and the 10 peaks of the lens: 1 = anterior capsule; 2 = anterior zone of disjunction; 3 = anterior superficial cortex; 4 = anterior deep cortex; 5 = anterior supranuclear layer; 6 = anterior nucleus; 7 = posterior nucleus; 8 = posterior supranuclear layer; 9 = posterior cortex; 10 = posterior capsule.

The pupillary diameter not only influences the visibility of the posterior capsule, but also projects an invisible shadow on its peripheral parts [10] such that an artificial density decrease of the posterior capsule begins at a certain distance from the optical axis, i.e. in the periphery [5]. This effect is of minor importance for the anterior capsule. To get an insight into the spatial density distribution of the capsules on both surfaces of the lens in normal subjects as well as the changes of this parameter during ageing and cataract development, we evaluated Scheimpflug images of 2 different meridians with multilinear microdensitometry.

Material and Methods

Scheimpflug images recorded with the Topcon SL-45 on Kodak T-Max 400 film from 25 patients in an age range between 19 and 63 years have been chosen for this study. The images of meridians 0° and 45° were evaluated on a Joyce Loebl microdensitometer applying multilinear microdensitometry [6]. A measurement window of 50 × 500 µm was moved upwards and downwards in parallel steps as shown in figure 1. Scan 0 corresponds to the optical axis of the eye (= rotating axis of the camera), +2 to +8 are parallel measurement planes below the optical axis, whereas −2 to −8 represent those above it. The lens density data have been individually normalized to corneal density. From each densitometric scan, peaks 1 and 10 have been chosen for calculation (fig. 2). The density data obtained are plotted against distance from the optical axis of the lens.

Results

Normal and cataractous lenses from patients in an age range between 22 and 58 years are presented. The density data for the capsules of the right and left lens are plotted sepa-

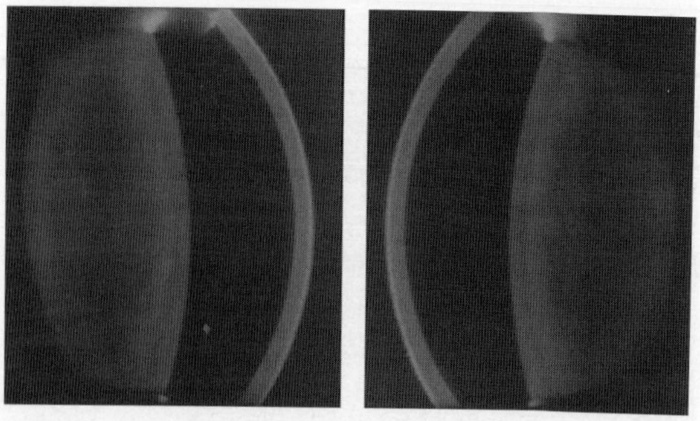

Fig. 3. 22-year-old normal case. The two meridians of the anterior (upper lines) and posterior capsules (lower lines) follow the same trend on both sides. Black line above = 45°; dotted line below = 45°. The density of the posterior capsule is generally lower than that of the anterior capsule.

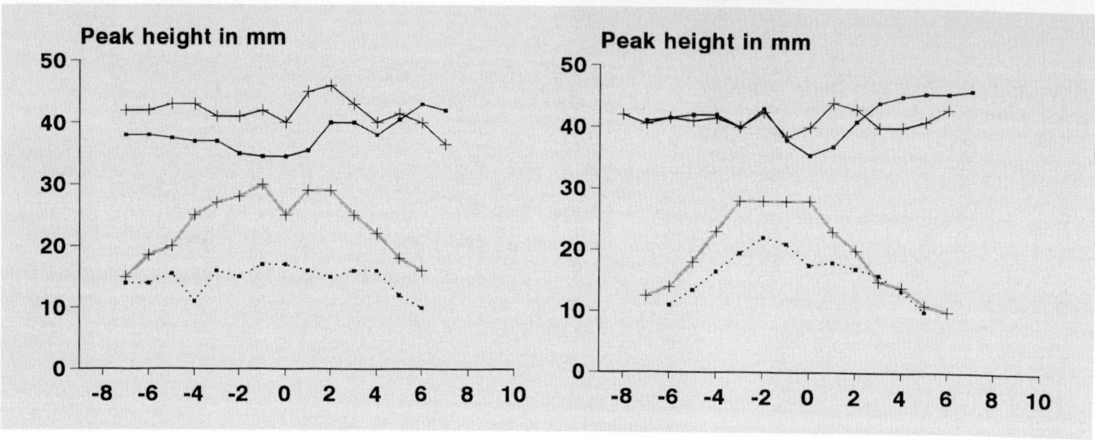

rately. The graphs in figure 3 contain, as an example, the data for the anterior and posterior capsules from the 2 meridians (0°, 45°). As a general observation, the density of the anterior capsule is higher than that of the posterior capsule (fig. 3–5) in normal subjects.

In younger cases, it could be demonstrated that the density of the anterior capsule, which is more or less uniform in the periphery, decreases in the area of the optical axis, perhaps due to the anterior sutural gap underneath. The density of the posterior capsule, however, always increases towards the center, sometimes with an indentation of the curve right in the axis. This again is possibly due to the sutural gap underneath. Furthermore, the anterior capsule obviously becomes more homogenous with age (fig. 4, 5). The posterior capsule keeps its trend to increase towards the axis (fig. 5). Especially the density data for the posterior capsule demonstrate the influence of the shadowing effect, as they always sharply decrease towards the periphery. This trend also becomes more pronounced with age, which again points to the influence of mydriasis especially on the posterior capsule, although there is also an effect on the periphery of the anterior capsule (fig. 5, 6).

The 58-year-old case with a posterior subcapsular cataract (fig. 6) not only shows a marked density increase in the cataractous area, which surpasses the density of the anterior capsule, but also demonstrates that the density of the normal anterior capsule increases with age (fig. 6). Its mean density increases by about 20%.

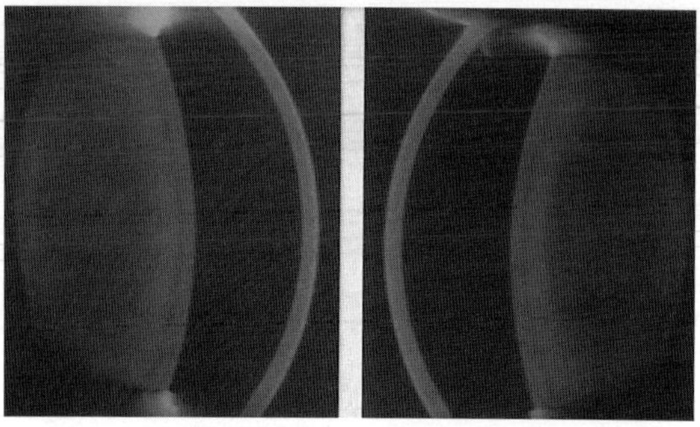

Fig. 4. 31-year-old normal case. Similar trends for the anterior and posterior capsules on both eyes.

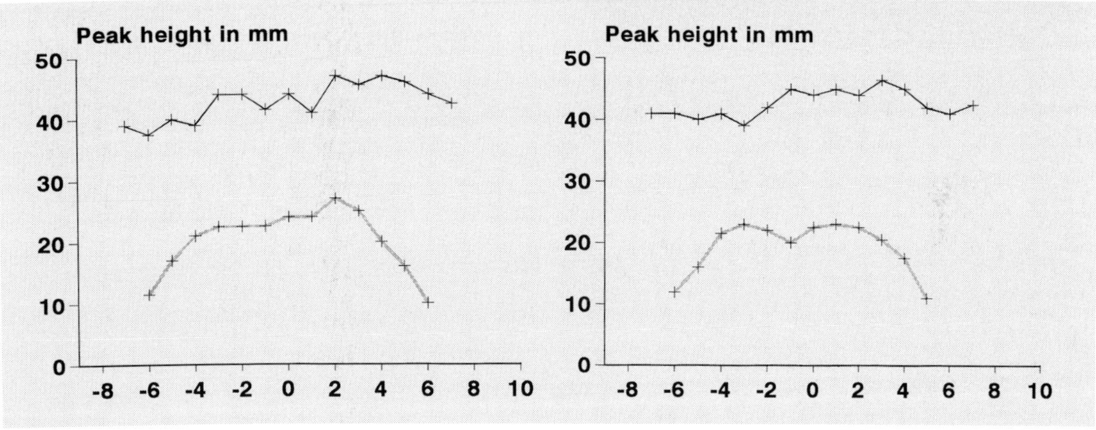

Conclusion

In general, it has been shown that the anterior capsule is always more dense in normal subjects than the posterior. This reflects the difference in thickness between both, but also potentially a difference in density of the capsular collagen packing. In addition, the anterior capsule is under lower tension than the posterior due to the underlying epithelium and the posterior capsule is permanently stretched during lens growth by fiber cell differentiation. An exception from this rule was a case of a posterior subcapsular cataract in a 58-year-old patient, where the density in the cataractous area at the posterior capsule was higher than that of the anterior capsule. In comparing between both surface lines with respect to homogeneity, the anterior capsule demonstrated a larger variation in density than the posterior capsule. There was no obvious trend for capsular density between the center and the periphery, but a clear trend for an increase of the anterior capsular density with age.

The posterior capsule in younger cases, in contrast, did show a trend in that the central part is more dense than the periphery. A few cases also showed a small indentation right in the axis, which most probably corresponds to the posterior sutural gap. The two meridians 0° and 45° demonstrated the same trends in normal subjects but nevertheless were not superimposable. A preliminary evaluation of further meridians indicates a distinct 3-dimensional scattering profile, which needs further evaluation.

The sharp density decrease of the posterior capsule towards the periphery underlines the

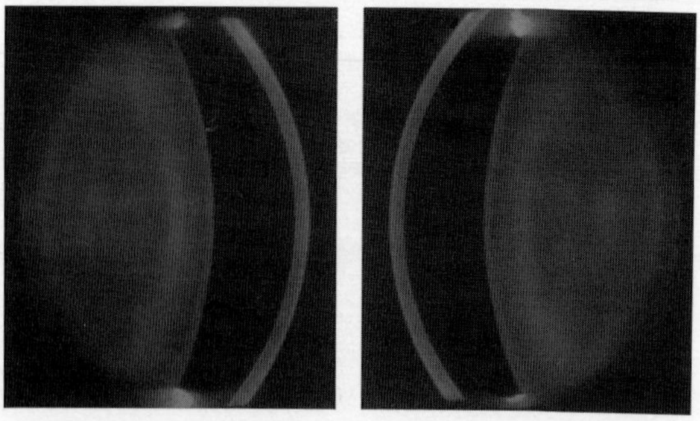

Fig. 5. 53-year-old normal case, similar trends for both capsules on both eyes.

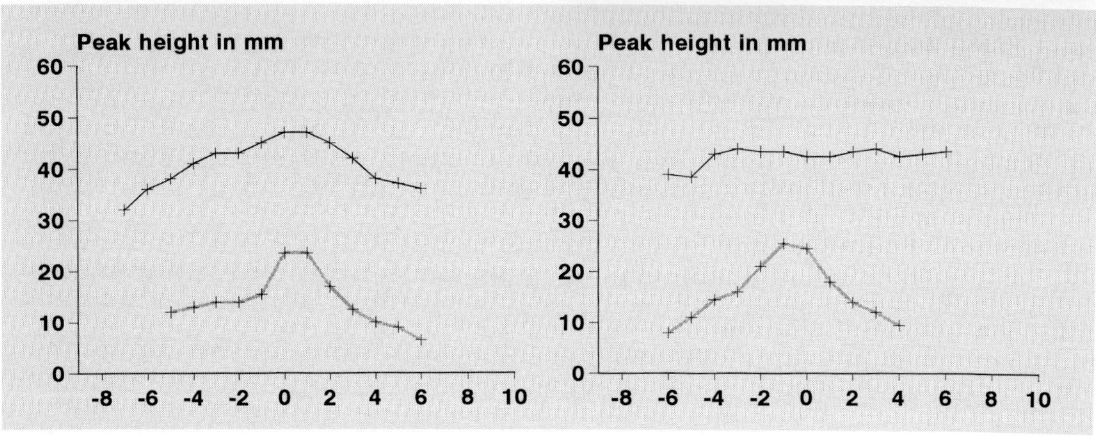

problem of the shadowing effect of the iris rim on the posterior capsule of the lens [9]. Considering the geometrical optical corrections for the real and virtual thickness of the lens established by Sparrow et al. [7], which are based on on-axis and off-axis measurements of the pupillary diameter and the ray tracing method for exact distortion compensation of the Scheimpflug image [8], it becomes obvious that a correction algorithm has to be introduced into the evaluation of the density of the posterior capsule to determine the extent of shadowing that influences the density data of its peripheral parts. Such an algorithm will be included into special image analytical software that is being developed by the authors.

Based on these corrections it will become possible to differentiate in older patients between presbyopia due to lack of lenticular accommodative capacity (changes in lens curvature due to increased thickness) and those changes due to an increase in light scattering of distinct regions of the lens during cataract development.

Calculation of the ratio of densities (peak heights) of the posterior/anterior capsules plotted against time provided a regression line that can be extrapolated to intersect the y-axis at 1. This demonstrates that it becomes possible to determine the normal protein-related density increase in different lens layers in relation to age.

Acknowledgements

The authors are indebted to Prof. Robert Weale from London and Dr. John Sparrow from Bristol for valuable discussions on this subject.

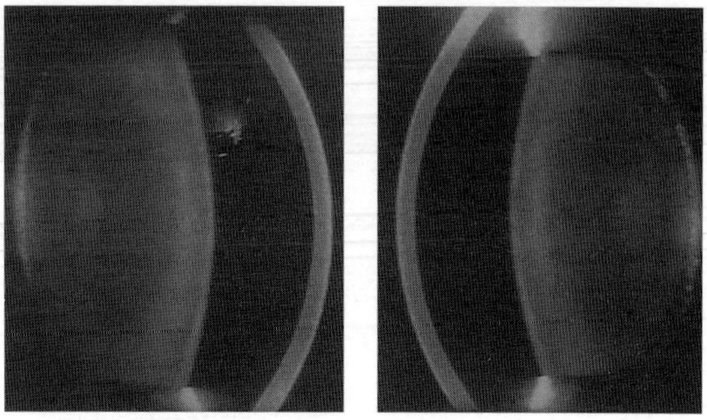

Fig. 6. 58-year-old case with posterior subcapsular cataracts on both eyes. Independently, the anterior capsule has increased in density due to aging.

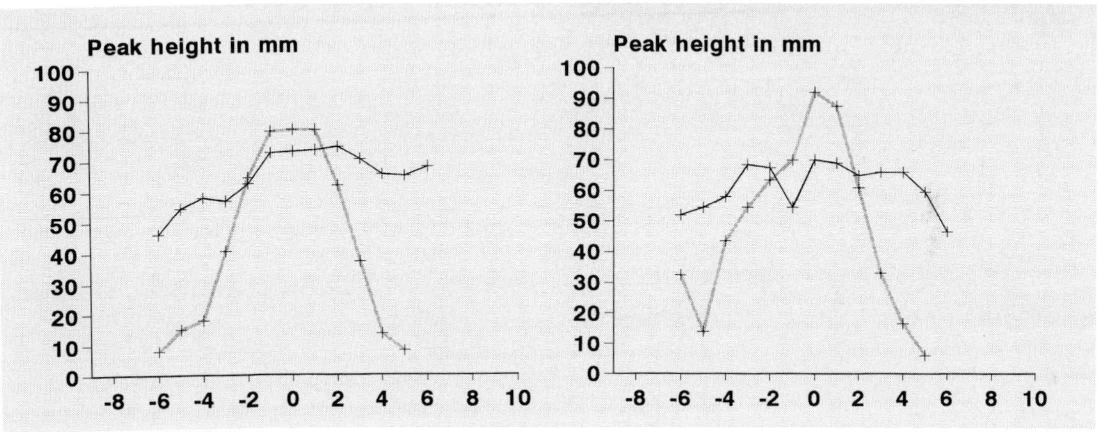

References

1 Drews C: Depth of field in slit lamp photography: An optical solution using the Scheimpflug principle. Ophthalmologica 1964;148:143–150.

2 Brown NAP: An advanced slit-image camera. Br J Ophthal 1972; 56:624–631.

3 Dragomirescu V, Hockwin O, Koch H-R, Sasaki K: Development of a new equipment for slit image photography according to Scheimpflug's principle. Interdiscipl Top Gerontol 1978;13:118–130.

4 Hockwin O, Lerman S, Laser H, Dragomirescu V: Image analysis of Scheimpflug photos of the lens by multiple linear microdensitometry. Lens Res 1985;2:337–350.

5 Mayer H: Habilitationsschrift, 11–15, Tübingen, 1986.

6 Hockwin O, Laser H, Kapper K: Image analysis of Scheimpflug negatives. Ophthalmic Res 1985;20:99–105.

7 Sparrow JM, Brown NAP, Bron AJ: Estimation of the thickness of the crystalline lens from on-axis and off-axis Scheimpflug photographs. Ophthal Physiol Opt 1993;13:291–294.

8 Kampfer T, Wegener A, Dragomirescu V, Hockwin O: Improved biometry of the anterior eye segment. Ophthalmic Res 1989;21: 239–248.

9 Mütze K: ABC der Optik. Hanau, Dausien, 1975.

10 Niesel P: Probleme der Spaltlampenphotographie der menschlichen Linse. Doc Ophthal 1966;20:131–140.

Ophthalmic
Research

Ophthalmic Res 1996;28(suppl 2):92–101

Ying Bo Shui
Masami Kojima
Kazuyuki Sasaki

Department of Ophthalmology,
Kanazawa Medical University,
Uchinada, Japan

A New Steroid-Induced Cataract Model in the Rat: Long-Term Prednisolone Applications with a Minimum of X-Irradiation

Key Words
Steroid cataract
Brown-Norway rat
Prednisolone acetate
X-irradiation
Scheimpflug photography
Image analysis
Cocataractogenesis

Abstract
In order to induce experimental steroid cataracts in rat eyes similar morphologically to those seen in human eyes, prednisolone acetate was administered either topically or systemically for 12 months with a low dose of X-irradiation as a cocataractogenic factor. Twenty-seven Brown-Norway rats were randomly divided into a control group (group I) with no steroid administration; an eyedrop group (group II) with a daily 1% prednisolone acetate instillation of a total volume of 1.0 mg/kg in both eyes, and a systemic group (group III) with a daily intramuscular injection of 0.8–1.0 mg/kg prednisolone acetate. The right eyes of animals in each group were X-irradiated with a single dose of 2 Gy. Topical and systemic steroid administrations started 2 weeks after X-irradiation. Anterior segment changes were documented with a slitlamp microscope and an anterior eye segment analysis system once a month. Body weight and blood glucose levels were examined every week and every 2 weeks, respectively. The mortality rates in groups I, II and III were 0, 11 (1/9) and 25% (3/12), respectively. The both lenses in group I showed a gradual increase in light-scattering intensity in the nuclear and supranuclear regions over time. Initial lens changes in both steroid-treated groups were Y-suture dissociation and a slight increase in light-scattering intensity in the posterior supranuclear region 3 months after prednisolone administration. Opacification of the anterior shallow cortex and the posterior subcapsular layer was observed after 10 months. X-irradiated eyes showed more prominent lens opacification as compared with nonirradiated eyes after 10 months in both group II and group III. Either topical or systemic administrations of prednisolone acetate over a long term successfully induced morphological lenticular changes in the rat similar to those found in human steroid-induced cataracts. A low dose of X-irradiation effectively accelerated opacification as a cocataractogenic risk. This new model will allow future investigation of steroid cataracts.

KARGER

E-Mail karger@karger.ch
Fax + 41 61 306 12 34
http://www.karger.ch

© 1996 S. Karger AG, Basel
0030–3747/96/0288–0092$10.00/0

Ying Bo Shui, MD
Department of Ophthalmology
Kanazawa Medical University
Uchinada, Ishikawa, 920-02 (Japan)

Introduction

Among human cataracts, steroid-induced posterior subcapsular cataract has been known as a typical iatrogenic ocular disease. Although in the majority of cases this type of cataract has been induced by systemic administration of steroids, topical steroid administration has rarely led to cataract [1–6]. In order to clarify the mechanism of steroid-induced cataract in human eyes, numerous attempts have been made to induce the same type of cataract in animals. Although topical or systemic corticosteroid administration has been mostly unsuccessful in inducing 'typical' cataracts, some authors have shown promising results, such as lens opacification in chick embryos and posterior subcapsular cataracts in rabbits [7–9]. Despite their morphological differences in comparison to human steroid-induced cataracts, these findings suggested that it may be possible to induce experimental cataract by steroids.

Steroid-induced cataracts in human eyes show nearly the same morphological lenticular changes even with different causative background states. However, patients who have received steroid either topically or systemically are usually not in a healthy state and must be considered as compromised hosts. This suggests that the desired experimental cataract in rat eyes might be induced or accelerated by co- and/or syncataractogenic factors [10]. The present study was based on recent investigations concerning intralenticular prednisolone acetate distribution in rabbit eyes [11] and light-scattering changes in different lenticular layers with a combination prednisolone administration and X-irradiation of 2 Gy in Brown-Norway rat eyes [12]. Given these preliminary observations, the authors attempted to follow lenticular changes for 1 year.

Materials and Methods

Animals

Twenty-seven 6-week-old male Brown-Norway rats (Sankyo Labo Service Co. Inc., Japan) were used in the experiments. The lenticular transparency and corneal conditions of all the rats were examined using the slit-lamp microscope (Topcon SL-5D) and documented by an anterior eye segment analysis system (Nidek EAS-1000) before starting the experiments [12]. The rats were maintained in a 12-hour light/dark cycle. Room temperature was kept at 25 ± 2 °C and humidity at 55 ± 3%. The rats were fed commercially available chow and given tap water ad libitum. The air was exchanged through an air filter system.

X-Irradiation

The right eyes of all rats were X-irradiated with a single dose of 2 Gy under anesthesia with 50 mg/kg i.p. of pentobarbital (Sankyo). Each rat was fixed on a turntable rotating 2 times/min during X-irradiation for 168 s (Sofron, BST 1505, 150 kV, 5 mA). The irradiated source came from the upper side of the rat head. The focal distance was 300 mm. The entire body of the rat except the right eye area was shielded by a specially designed zinc protector [12].

Steroid Administration

Twenty-seven rats were randomly divided into three groups. Six rats (group I) were observed throughout the examination without drug administration. The eyes of nine rats (group II) were instilled daily with 10 μl of a 1% prednisolone acetate ophthalmic solution (Santen Pharmaceutical Co.) into the cul-de-sac 2 times at 15-min intervals. Twelve rats (group III) were administered 0.8–1.0 mg/kg i.m. of a 1% prednisolone acetate suspension (Shionogi Pharmaceutical Co.) daily. Steroid applications to groups II and III started 2 weeks after X-irradiation. In order to observe the animals for as long as possible, the above doses of steroid were sometimes gradually reduced when the health of the rats deteriorated, and the doses of prednisolone acetate were returned to normal after recovery of rats.

Observation of the Anterior Eye Segment

Changes in the anterior part of the rat eyes including the cornea and the lens were observed once a month through a slitlamp microscope and recorded by an anterior eye segment analysis system [13] under dilation of the pupils by a 1% atropine solution. One photographer, who was blind to the treatment of the animals, took all the Scheimpflug and retroillumination images. Following the authors' previous method,

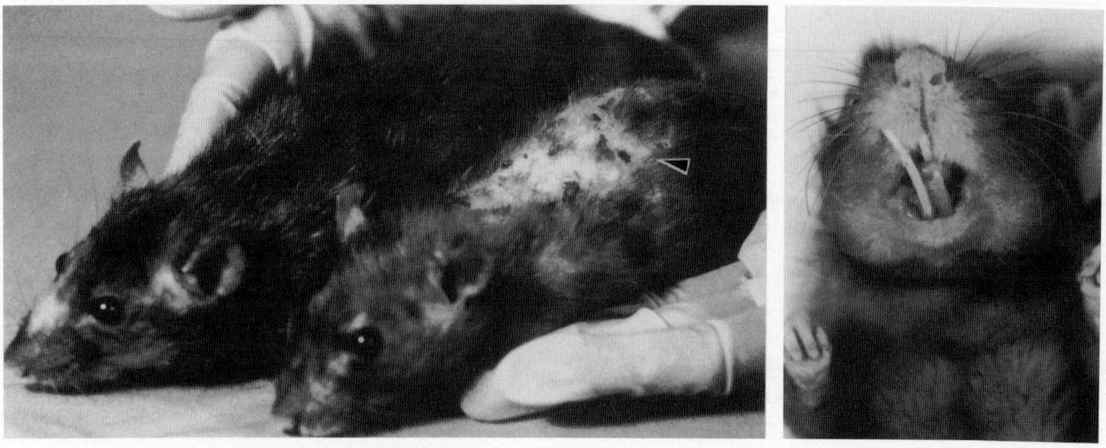

A B

Fig. 1. A The difference in fur between the rats of group I (left) and those of group III (right). The hair of group-III rats showed serious loss and faded color. The arrowhead points out the area of a former skin ulcer. **B** Rat teeth with abnormal growth in length in group III.

changes in lenticular transparency were quantitatively evaluated by determination of light-scattering intensity and application of a modified program for opaque-area measurement of lenticular retroillumination images [12, 14]. The observations were performed over a period of 12 months.

General Health Examination

Rat body weights and blood glucose levels were examined once a week and every 2 weeks, respectively. Blood glucose was measured through tail vein blood by a commercially available instrument (Glutest E®, Sanwa) under nonfasting conditions. Characteristics of their skin, hair, activity and teeth were also checked weekly.

Statistical Analyses

All of the experimental data were evaluated using a two-tailed t test. p values less than 0.05 were considered significant.

Results

General Condition

Although some rats died during the observation period, the survival ratios were 100% (6/6) in group I, and 89% (8/9) and 75% (9/12) in groups II and III, respectively. All of the group-I rats maintained an almost healthy condition except for a slight loss of hair on the head. The rats of group II showed mild hair loss on the body and faded hair color. A few rats of group II had local skin ulcers for a short time. The rats in group III showed prominent hair loss on their whole bodies and, in particular, markedly faded hair color. Some of them formed skin ulcers, which recovered without any special treatment after a temporary reduction of the dose of prednisolone acetate administration. Four rats were housed together in the same cage, and the rats in group III had more severe fights compared to the other two groups. Only in group III some of the rats' teeth (3/12) became fragile, broke, or showed abnormal growth, which interfered with food intake (fig. 1).

Body Weight

The body weight of the group-I rats showed a normal increasing pattern during the observation period. Group II showed a significant inhibition of the body weight increase after 10

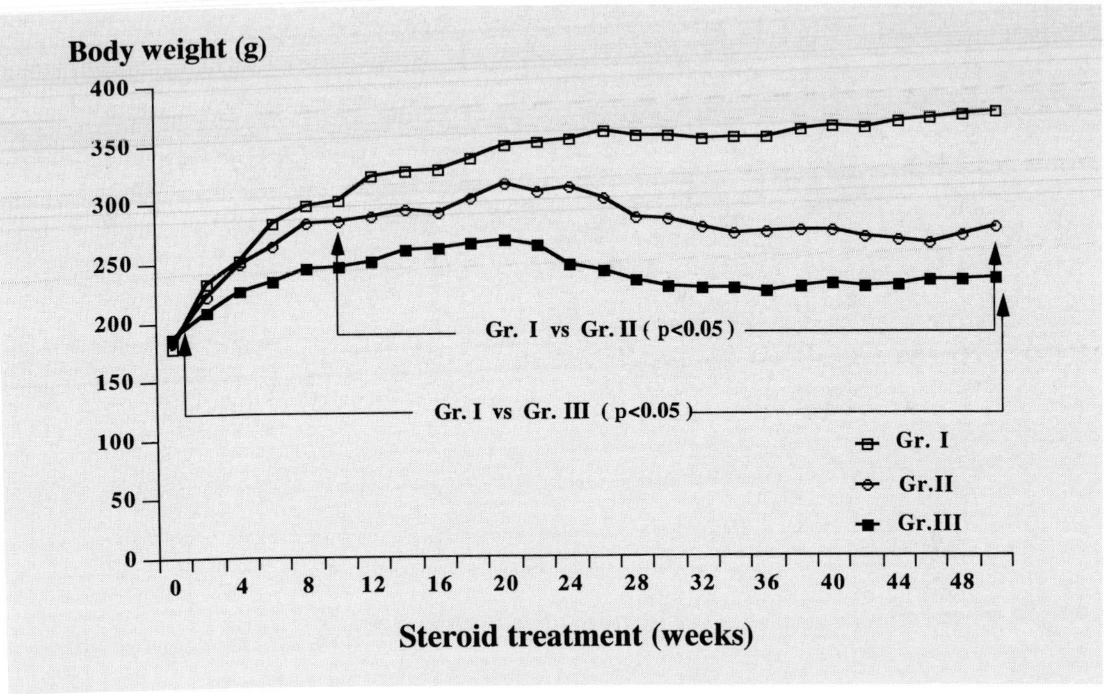

Fig. 2. Body weight changes in the three groups. Significantly different ranges are joined by brackets with arrowheads and p values are indicated.

weeks of steroid eyedrop application as compared with the group-I rats ($p < 0.05$). An inhibition of body weight increase with ageing in group III was noticed from the first week of steroid treatment as compared with group I ($p < 0.05$). The above tendencies lasted in groups II and III until the end of the observation period (fig. 2).

Blood Glucose Level

The mean values of the blood glucose level in the three groups were within the normal range (3.79–5.35 mmol/l) throughout the observation period (fig. 3). However, that of group III showed a temporary increase of the blood glucose level compared with groups I and II from the 10th to the 30th week ($p < 0.05$). No sign of steroid-induced diabetes was found during the observation period.

Lenticular Changes

The lenticular changes induced by corticosteroid were slow in the first half year of the 12-month experimental period. There were no macroscopical significant differences in light-scattering in the lens layers among the three groups at the beginning of the 3rd month. However, quantitative evaluation of the opaque area by lenticular retroillumination image analysis showed significantly increased opaque values in the right eyes of groups II and III compared with the right eyes of group I from 3 months onwards. The changes became constant from the 7th month and accelerated from the 10th month. Among the two prednisolone-treated groups, group-II eyes finally showed more prominent changes than those of group III (fig. 4). Alterations in the lenticular opaque area of the left eyes (no

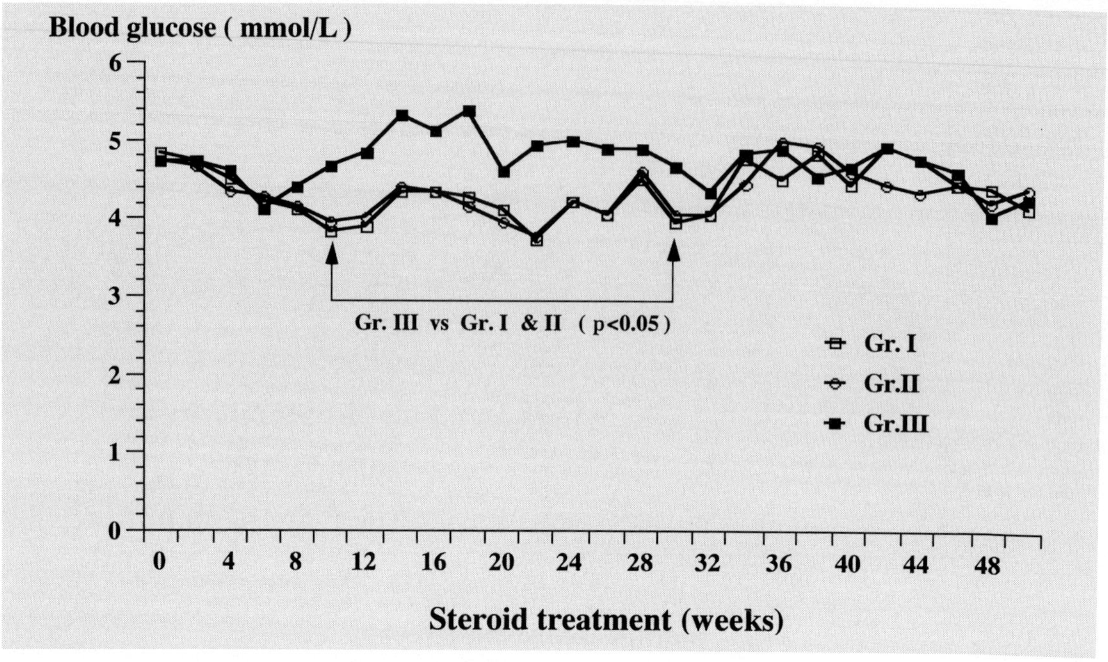

Fig. 3. Blood glucose changes in the three groups.

X-irradiation) is shown in figure 5. The first significant increase of the opaque area occurred in the 2nd month of the topical steroid treatment. The same change appeared in the systemic group from the 4th month. Again, the lenticular opacities accelerated from the 10th month in the same way as in the irradiated right eyes. Although the opaque lenticular areas showed a tendency to be slightly larger in the X-irradiated right eyes than in the nonirradiated left eyes, there was no statistical significance between both eyes in the steroid-treated groups except during the last 2 months. In group I, there was no significant difference between the right and left eyes throughout the observation time.

In both prednisolone-treated eyes, the initial macroscopically detectable changes, such as Y-suture dissociation and prominent increase of light-scattering intensity in the posterior supranuclear region, were noticed after 3 months of prednisolone application. A half-moon-shaped opacity surrounding the posterior embryonic nucleus was seen in some eyes of groups II and III. These changes slowly and constantly increased with time. A faint string-like opacity in the anterior lenticular cortex first appeared in some animals of groups II and III from the 8th month. Table 1 indicates the incidence and time of the appearance of this opacity in the anterior cortex. Thereafter, opaque dots and vacuoles were noticed along with the posterior suture line. They gradually expanded, and posterior subcapsular cataracts developed approximately 10 months after steroid administration (fig. 6). Table 2 shows the incidence and time of onset of posterior subcapsular opacity development. This change was particularly dominant in group II compared with group III. Also, group III

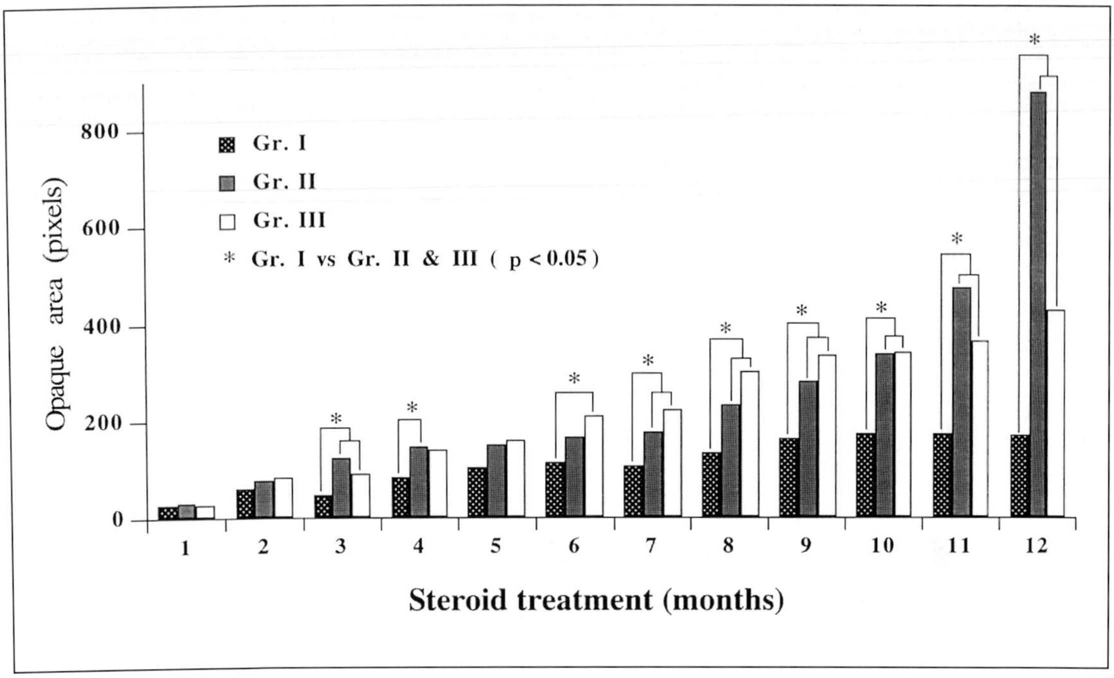

Fig. 4. Lenticular opaque area changes in the X-irradiated right eyes in the three groups. Bars represent the mean pixel values.

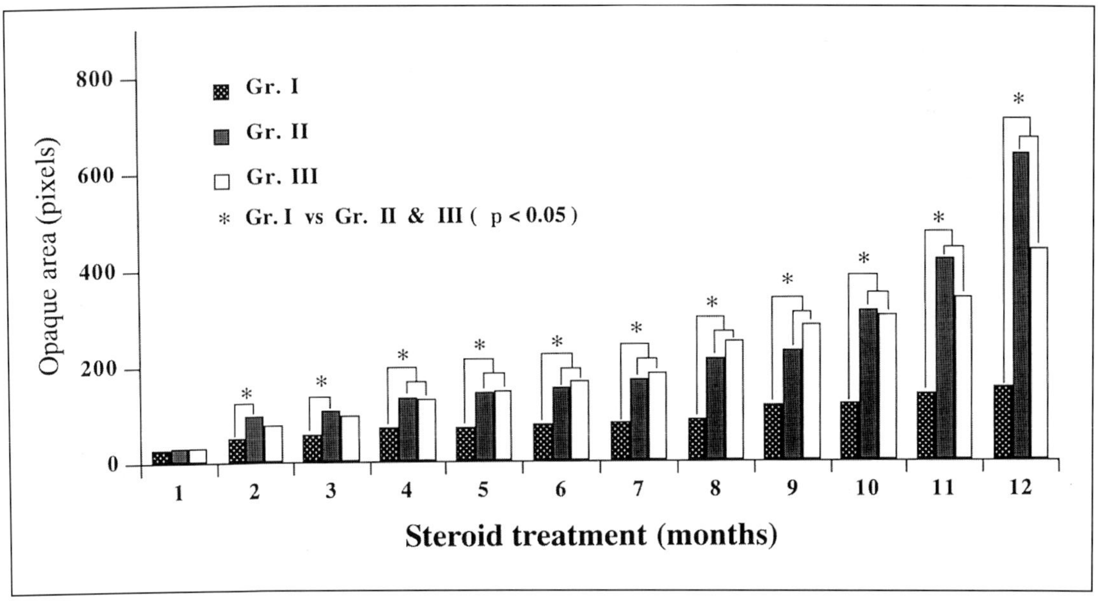

Fig. 5. Lenticular opaque area changes in the non-X-irradiated left eyes in the three groups. Bars represent the mean pixel values.

Table 1. The incidence and time of onset of anterior cortical opacification

Months	Right eyes			Left eyes		
	group I	group II	group III	group I	group II	group III
8	0/6	3/9	3/12	0/6	0/9	0/12
9	1/6	6/8[1]	6/12	0/6	0/9	1/12
10	3/6	8/8[1]	9/11[2]	0/6	3/9	2/11[2]
11	3/6	8/8[1]	10/11[2]	0/6	5/9	3/11[2]
12	4/6	6/6[1, 2]	8/9[2]	0/6	8/8[1, 2]	8/9[2]

[1] Numbers omitted when the lens could not be observed completely through the cornea.
[2] Numbers omitted when rats died.

Table 2. The incidence and time of onset of posterior subcapsular opacity development

Months	Right eyes			Left eyes		
	group I	group II	group III	group I	group II	group III
8	0/6	0/9	0/12	0/6	0/9	0/12
9	0/6	0/8[1]	0/12	0/6	0/9	0/12
10	0/6	5/8[1]	2/11[2]	0/6	2/9	0/11[2]
11	0/6	8/8[1]	6/11[2]	0/6	3/9	2/11[2]
12	1/6	6/6[1, 2]	8/9[2]	0/6	6/8[1, 2]	5/9[2]

[1] Numbers omitted when the lens could not be observed completely through the cornea.
[2] Numbers omitted when rats died.

showed more individual differences during cataract formation. Although the morphological changes of the lens of the right eye were more serious than those in the left eyes in both steroid-treated groups, their incidence were almost the same. It was not possible to document all lenses after the 10th month of steroid application because of the corneal disorders.

Scheimpflug slitlamp images revealed a slight increase in light-scattering intensity on the fetal nuclei of the lens with ageing in group I with and without X-irradiation; however, the intensity seemed to be higher in the right eyes with X-irradiation than in the nonirradiated left eyes. In group-I rats, there was a faint string-like opacification, which was first seen in a limited area of the anterior cortex 9 months after the start of this experiment, with a few opaque dots occurring on the posterior suture line. These findings progressed very slowly until the end of the observation period. No similar findings were seen in the non-X-irradiated left eyes.

Other ocular side effects, such as superficial punctate keratitis, were common in both steroid-treated groups. Corneal ectasia, corneal thinness, ulcer or rupture and leukoma formations occurred with a higher incidence

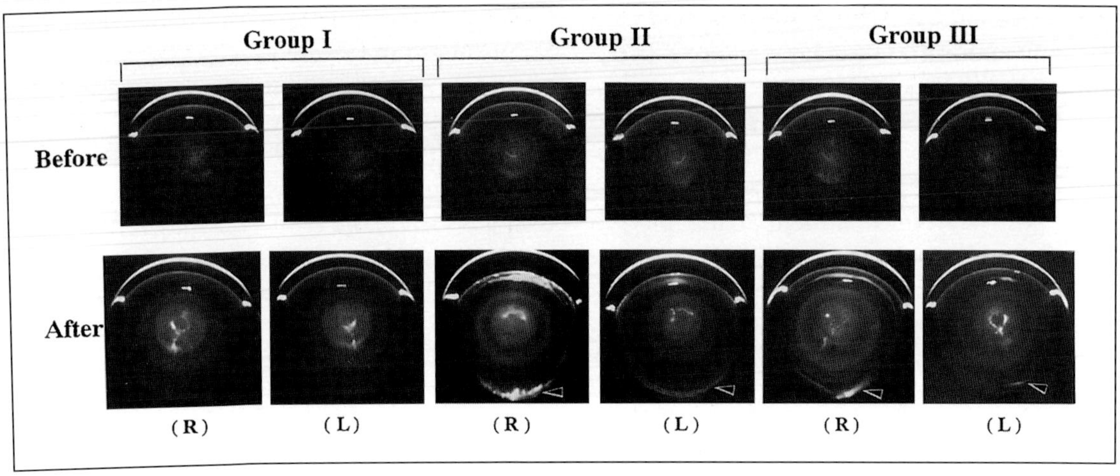

Fig. 6. EAS-1000 Scheimpflug images: the lens conditions in the three groups before the start of steroid administration and after the 1 year steroid treatment. R represents the right eyes, which received 2 Gy X-irradiation. L represents the left eyes, which were shielded from the X-ray. Arrowheads indicate the posterior cortical opacities in groups II and III.

in group II (50% of eyes) than group III (8%). There were no special findings on the corneas of group I.

Discussion

Steroid-induced cataract is well known as a typical iatrogenic disease in ophthalmology. As yet, no suitable drugs have replaced corticosteroids, and a large number of clinical cases still require the application of corticosteroids to alleviate or inhibit disease progression. However, since of the several types of cataract the cause of the steroid-induced cataract is known, its occurrence or progression should be preventable. Yet the mechanisms of steroid-induced cataracts have not been sufficiently clarified. For this purpose, many investigations have been performed by previous authors [15] attempting to mimic the cataract seen in humans, but the results are still far from ideal. We hypothesize that previous experiments failed because the animals used were not able to survive for the long observation period. In addition, no reliable and advanced experimental methodology for objective estimation of cataractous changes as applied in this study was used in previous studies.

To explore the appropriate approach for this investigation, a pharmacokinetic study on prednisolone was performed first to investigate whether steroids, administered either topically or systemically, penetrate the lens [11]. The majority of such studies of intralenticular drug dynamics performed previously used whole-lens material and the obtained data were either negative or below the detectable steroid dose. The methodology applied here was a microsectioning technique by which regional penetration of the administered drugs was detectable in the lens. The present authors knew the topographic distribution of prednisolone in rabbit eyes from the results obtained by the above methods. With the eyedrop administration method, the drug penetrated more easily into the lens than with retrobulbar or intramuscular injections. In accordance with these data, two of the most regular and simple clinic methods, the eyedrop and the intramuscular injection of prednisolone, were applied in this long-term experiment with steroid treatment. The in vivo experimental results showed that the incidence of cataract formation and time schedule were higher in group II than in group III. This indicates that steroid-induced cataract formation is strongly related to steroidal concentration in the lens, and the steroid itself may have some direct influence on lenticular opacification.

Steroid-induced cataracts in humans show the following characteristics: usually, the incidence of steroid-related side effects correlates with the dosage, duration of therapy, age, route of administration and underlying disease [16]. Among the above characteristics, the authors considered that particularly the immunocompromised host is at a greater risk for steroid-induced cataract. Therefore, this study aimed at inducing steroid cataract in rats with an abnormal health condition, while other previous attempts used animals with a completely normal background. This meant that the administered corticosteroid might act as a co-cataractogenic or syncataractogenic agent with a limited exposure area and quite a low dose of X-irradiation. For long-term observation of the course of lenticular changes, prednisolone acetate, one of the steroids usually suggested for long-term application, was selected. Furthermore, as it is difficult for animals to tolerate high doses of systemic corticosteroid for a long-term follow-up study, we used steroid dosages that were close to clinical applications [17] and dosages readjusted appropriately according to the animals' general health.

Both steroid-treated groups, II and III, showed the similar tendencies in lenticular changes until the 10th month of prednisolone therapy. Interestingly, at that time the alterations in group II were accelerated and aggravated to anterior and posterior opacities. The anterior cortical opacity appeared to be more prominent in the right eyes than in the left eyes in groups II and III. The lenticular changes seen in the right eyes may reflect a co- and/or syncataractogenic cataract formation even though no statistically significant difference could be found between the X-irradiated and nonirradiated eyes except during the last 2 months.

The lenticular changes in group I appeared in some right eyes that received 2 Gy X-irradiation, with a slight string-like opacity located on the anterior cortex and a few opaque dots on the posterior suture line 9 months after X-irradiation. The left eyes seemed normal by in vivo observation. Low-dose X-ray only interfered with vision to a small degree or not at all after a 1-year latent period.

The body growth of group-III rats showed a significant inhibition from the first week of steroid treatment. The overall physical condition, such as marked hair loss, skin ulcer, teeth disorders and a 25% mortality rate, corresponds with known side effects found in humans [17]. Abnormal growth in the teeth was probably related to osteoporosis. Blood glucose levels remained within a normal range in all three groups during the experimental period. However, there was a period of significant elevation of blood glucose from the 10th to the 30th week in group III, which received systemic steroid administration. This might have been caused by increasing gluconeogenesis and decreasing cellular sensitivity to insulin. This reaction was not severe enough to aggravate diabetes as previously reported [7] and resolved later. Considerable systemic absorption of topical prednisolone acetate was observed, especially with long-term instillation. Rosenblum et al. [18] reported that 20–35% of topically administered dexamethasone was found systemically in rabbits 24 h after instillation. Our previous study of prednisolone penetration also showed that a 0.1% prednisolone acetate ophthalmic solution could be detected in rabbit serum after its instillation for a long term [11]. The present study showed a significant inhibition in growth induced by topical steroid application after 10 weeks of treatment. Even though other systemic side effects were fewer than in the injection group, the topical side effects, such as superficial punctate keratitis, corneal ectasia, corneal thinness, ulcer or rupture and leukoma formations, were more serious in the topical group than in the systemic group.

Although it is premature to conclude that the newly established model in this investigation is exactly the same as the steroid-induced cataracts seen in human eyes, the authors suggest that it may be quite close to the human steroid cataract and believe that it will be a recommendable model to clarify the mechanisms of steroid-induced cataracts in future.

Acknowledgements

The authors are grateful to Professor Kawarai, Department of Anatomy, Professor Imanishi, Department of Physiology, and Visiting Professor Hockwin, Department of Ophthalmology, Kanazawa Medical University, for their valuable advice. The support of the Welfare Ministry of Japan is gratefully acknowledged.

References

1 Black RL, Oglesby RB, von Sallmann L, Bunim JJ: Posterior subcapsular cataracts induced by corticosteroid in patients with rheumatoid arthritis. JAMA 1960;174:166–171.
2 Crews SJ: Posterior subcapsular lens opacities in patients on longterm corticosteroid therapy. Br Med J 1963;5346:1644–1647.
3 Sundmark E: The occurrence of posterior subcapsular cataracts in patients on long-term systemic corticosteroid therapy. Acta Ophthalmol 1963;41:515–523.
4 Valerio M: Les dangers de la corticonothérapie locale prolongée. Bull Mém Soc Fr Ophthalmol 1963;76: 572–580.
5 Frandsen E: Glaucoma and cataract as complications to topical steroid therapy. Acta Ophthalmol 1966;44: 307–312.
6 Cronin TP: Cataract with topical use of corticosteroid and idoxuridine. Arch Ophthalmol 1964;72: 198–199.
7 Tarkkanen A, Esilä R, Liesmaa M: Experimental cataracts following long-term administration of corticosteroids. Acta Ophthalmol 1966;44: 665–668.
8 Bucala R, Gallati M, Manabe S, Cotlier E, Cerami A: Glucocorticoid-lens protein abducts in experimentally induced steroid cataracts. Exp Eye Res 1985;40:853–863.
9 Nishigori H, Lee JW, Iwatsuru M: An animal model for cataract research: Cataract formation in developing chick embryo by glucocorticoid. Exp Eye Res 1983;36:617–622.
10 Hockwin O, Wegener A: Syn- and cocataractogenesis: A system for testing subliminal lens toxicity. Concepts Toxicol 1987;4:241–249.
11 Kojima M: Drug distribution studies in single lens layers through the application of a sectioning technique; in Weisse I, Hockwin O, Green K, Tripathi RC (eds): Ocular Toxicology. New York, Plenum Press, 1995, pp 121–134.
12 Shui Y, Kojima M, Hockwin O, Sasaki K: In vivo morphological changes in rat lenses induced by the administration of prednisolone after subliminal X-irradiation. A preliminary report. Ophthalmic Res 1995; 27(3):178–186.
13 Kojima M, Sasaki K: Application of a new Scheimpflug camera (EAS-1000) to animal cataract models. Ophthalmol Res 1992;24:3–9.
14 Sasaki K, Sakamoto Y, Shibata T, Emori Y: A new anterior èye segment analysis system. Ophthalmic Res 1990;22(suppl):3–8.
15 Urban RC, Cotlier E: Corticosteroid-induced cataracts. Surv Ophthalmol 1986;31:102–110.
16 Albert DM, Jakobiec FA, Robinson NL: Principles and Practice of Ophthalmology. Basic Sci. Philadelphia, Saunders, 1994, vol 4, pp 1013–1022.
17 American Medical Association: Drug Evaluations, ed 6. Philadelphia, Saunders, 1986, pp 1089–1104.
18 Rosenblum C, Dengler RE, Geoffroy RF: Ocular absorption of dexamethasone phosphate sodium by rabbit. Arch Ophthalmol 1967;77: 23.

Ophthalmic Research

Ophthalmic Res 1996;28(suppl 2):102–108

Viorel Dragomirescu[a]
Otto Hockwin[b,1]

[a] Remagen-Unkelbach, and
[b] University of Bonn, Germany

Rotating Slit Image Camera TOPCON SL 45

New Developments for Simultaneous Image Acquisition by Photographic and CCD-Assisted On-Line Documentation

Key Words
Slit image camera
Photographic imaging
On-line imaging
Combined photo and CCD imaging equipment
TOPCON SL 45 (new generation)
Scheimpflug color images
Lens endogenous fluorescence measurement

Abstract
In a first approach the photographic camera part of the SL 45 B has been replaced by a CCD camera (2/3″ black-and-white camera/Teli CS 3440 CCD B/W Tokyo Electronic Industry Co., Ltd.) unit thus enabling direct image acquisition and computer assisted analyses. Images have a full length of 8.8 mm. The images can be taken with only the observation light, no flash is necessary. Thus, the images can also be recorded on a VCR performing a complete rotation of the slit and all lens sections can be monitored obtaining almost three-dimensional information about the lens transparency/cataract formation. The further improvement is the on-line imaging for all SL-45 cameras in having CCD acquisition *together with* the usual 35-mm film photography. This is very important for the documentation of the lens coloration and for measuring lens fluorescence. For this TOPCON SL 45 (new generation) we are using the '2nd Scheimpflug condition' located within the eye piece of a SL 45 which is taken with a CS b/w No. 8310 C (Tokyo Electronic Industry Co., Ltd.). It is possible to integrate the CCD system in all TOPCON SL 45 Cameras (1st and 2nd production charge as well as SL 45 B).

Introduction

Scheimpflug imaging of the anterior eye section has been mainly achieved and supported by the construction of the TOPCON SL 45 [1]. Most of the developments for the use of this method in clinical and experimental eye research and investigations into the scope and limitations of this procedure were

[1] Visiting Professor, Department of Ophthalmology, Kanazawa Medical University, Uchinada, Japan.

KARGER

E-Mail karger@karger.ch
Fax + 41 61 306 12 34
http://www.karger.ch

© 1996 S. Karger AG, Basel
0030–3747/96/0288–0102$10.00/0

Prof. Dr. Otto Hockwin
Tulpenweg 4
D–53757 Sankt Augustin (Germany)

performed within the first 10 years after the industrial manufacturing of the TOPCON equipment [2–4].

Around 1980 [5], a new camera version of the Scheimpflug principle was developed by introducing the on-line imaging as demonstrated with the ZEISS SLC system. The on-line documentation with its rapid control of the image quality became more and more important, new equipment became available by the construction of the Oxford Camera System Case 2000 [6] and by the EAS 1000 NIDEK Camera [7]. The NIDEK equipment which permits also retroillumination imaging of the lens is at present the Scheimpflug-hardware of choice. A comparison of the TOPCON SL 45 with the NIDEK EAS 1000 demonstrated the advantages and limitations of both systems [8].

In order to obtain on-line documentation with the TOPCON SL 45 Huebscher and Schmidt [9] (with only a limited depth of the image) and Egner et al. [10] demonstrated the replacement of the photographic camera part by a CCD system.

The disadvantages of these new devices were the loss of the photographic imaging of the lens coloration [11, 12] as all CCDs used are monochrome. Moreover, the recording of the endogenous lens fluorescence became impossible [13]. Unfortunately, also the photoprints for teaching, publications and other demonstrations of on-line images taken from the screen were of poor quality. Many authors still used for this purpose the 'old' SL 45 photo-camera.[2]

We therefore looked into the possibility to reconstruct the SL 45 in a way to enable the traditional photographic imaging as well as the on-line documentation by a CCD camera. We here present the most modern equipment which can be used for all applications developed till now for the slit image documentation of the anterior eye segment according to Scheimpflug's principle including color images as well as measuring lens fluorescence.

Material and Methods

With a TOPCON SL 45 B, a first approach to on-line registration was made by removal of the camera part and fitting in this space a CCD Camera (2/3" black-and-white camera/Teli CS 3440 CCD B/W Tokyo Electronic Industry) unit. The image has a depth of 8.8 mm and covers the whole distance of the human anterior eye segment (cornea-anterior chamber-lens). The equipment is shown in figure 1; it is directly connected to the observation screen and to the computer system for data storage and image analysis (fig. 2). The image of the anterior eye segment obtained is demonstrated in figure 3 with the prints of image analysis for density readings at distinct sections of the lens.[3]

The main improvement of the SL 45 slit image camera was the additional on-line equipment saving the photographic documentation for the valuable techniques already mentioned. This was achieved by using the '2nd Scheimpflug image' of the viewfinder by introducing another half mirror, an additional lens system of f = 25 mm and the connection to a CCD b/w camera. For this we used a CS 8310 C of Tokyo Electronic Industry. The image sensor has 756 × 581 active pixels, the active image area is 8.8 × 6.6 mm (2/3") with 625 lines. The minimum sensitivity is reached with 0.5 lx.

The slit beam alignment to the patient's eye is controlled by the camera operator with the observation via viewfinder of the equipment which guarantees a high reproducibility of the imaging being superior to other ways of alignment. This is very important for repeated long-term patients control. It is also more favorable for all animal examinations with Scheimpflug equipment.

The diagram of this additional CCD camera installation into the SL 45 arrangement is demonstrated in

2 See LOGO of the 7th Scheimpflug Club Meeting, June 1995 at Kanazawa, Japan.

3 Evaluation by TOPCON software; we thank TOPCON Corporation, Tokyo and TOPCON Europe B.V. (Mr. P.J.W. Gelissen) for their valuable cooperation.

figure 4. Figure 5 shows the TOPCON SL 45 Photo/Video instrument. In figure 6, the viewfinder region with the location of the CCD part is demonstrated. On the upper left side of figure 6, the intact photo camera back can be seen.

Results

The TOPCON SL 45 permits an additional mounting of a CCD camera system, so that with the new version it becomes possible to obtain images of the anterior eye segment by photography as well as by on-line registration via an electronic camera. The obtained pictures demonstrated in figure 7a, b with a phantom eye and in figure 8a, b with a human volunteer (30 years old, without dilation of the iris!) were taken with flash illumination. Figures 7a and 8a are the photographs whereas 7b and 8b demonstrate the video images.

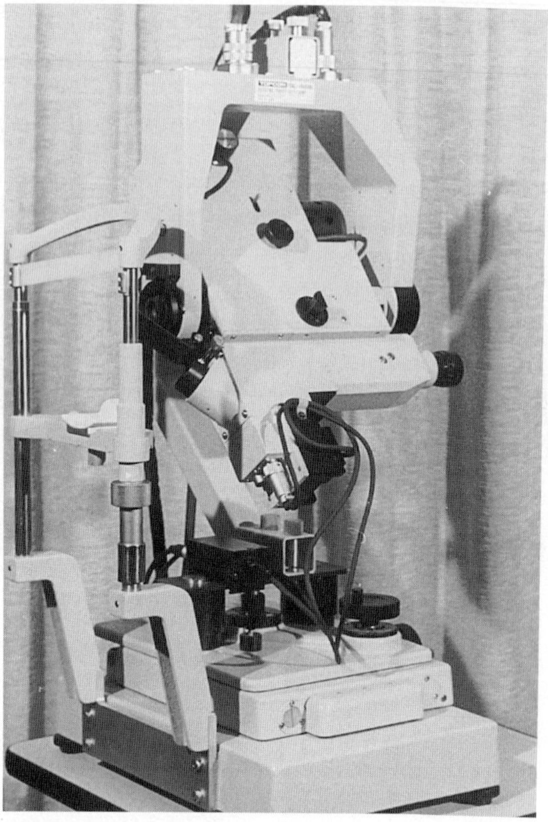

Fig. 1. TOPCON SL 45 B after removal of the photo camera back with attached CCD camera.

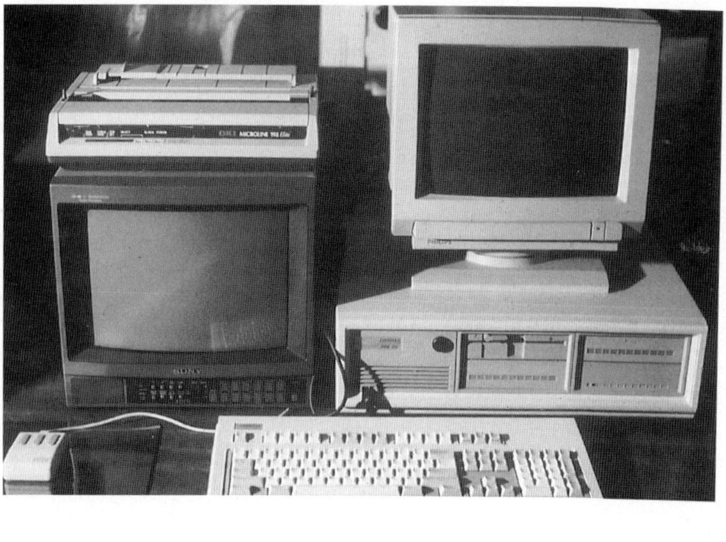

Fig. 2. Observation screen for the video imaging with the instrument shown in figure 1 and the computer system. The slit beam alignment to the patient's eye is controlled by the operator of the camera with help of the view finder.

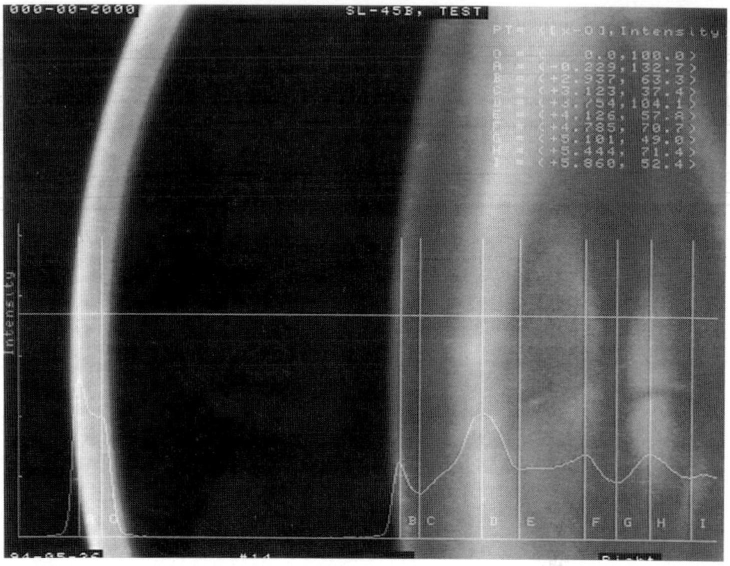

Fig. 3. Image analysis of cornea and several lens sections by computer assisted densitometric evaluation.

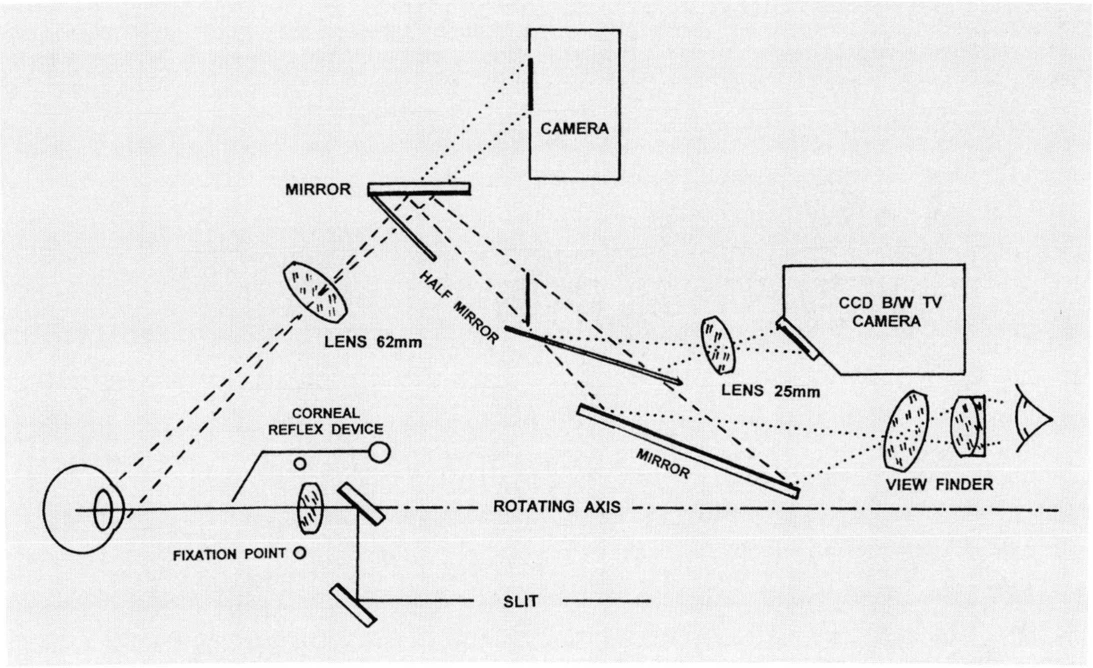

Fig. 4. Schematic drawing of the Topcon SL 45 modified for photography and video. Alignment of the camera is controlled in the viewfinder for both techniques using the observation light.

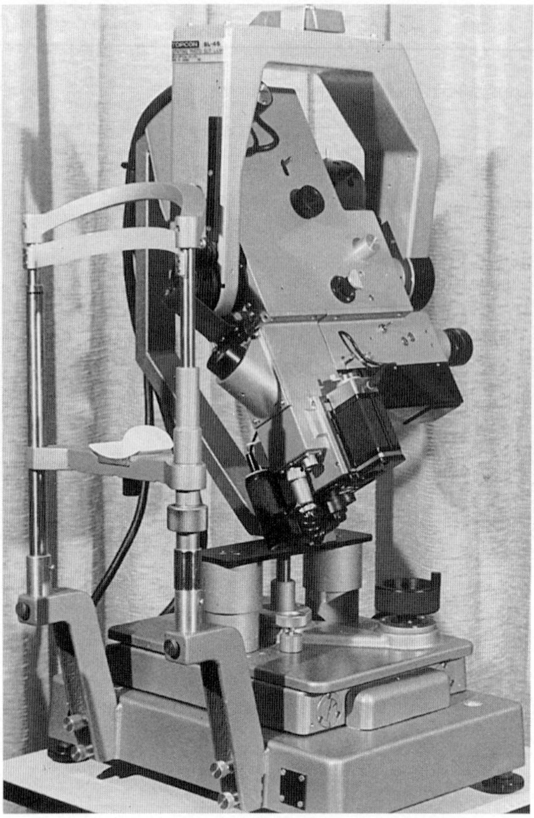

The sensitivity of the CCD system is very high, the illumination by the observation light of the SL 45 is completely enough for the on-line imaging. This has advantages for VCR recording while the slit beam is rotated. Herewith an almost three-dimensional information of the lens transparency/opacity condition is obtained.

Discussion

Constructing the highly approved rotating slit image camera TOPCON SL 45 as an instrument for documentation of the anterior eye segment by the (traditional) photographic method and simultaneously with the on-line image by a CCD camera a new device for application of the Scheimpflug technique to

Fig. 5. Topcon SL 45 with traditional photo camera and with additional CCD camera for on-line imaging.

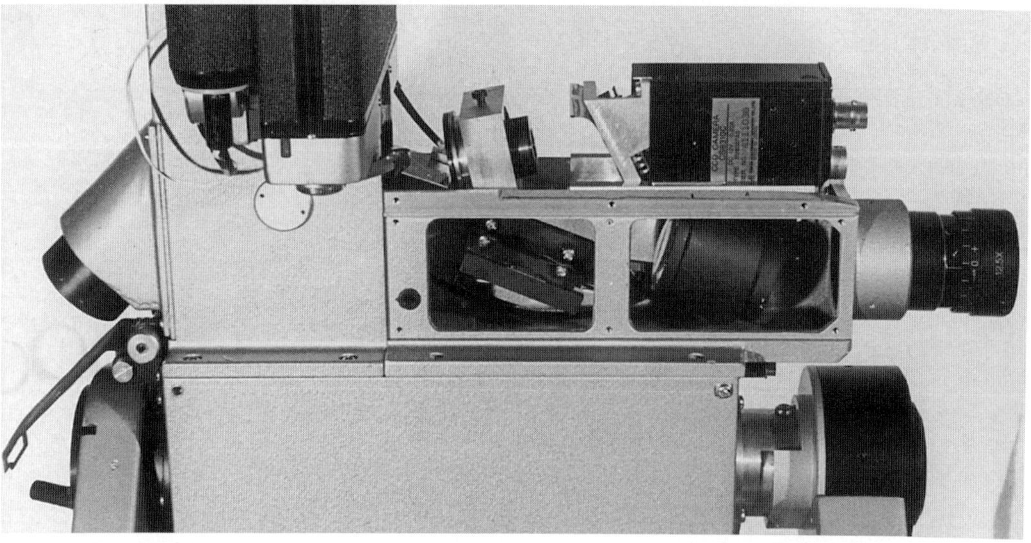

Fig. 6. Location of the additional CCD camera behind the original photo camera back and above the view finder.

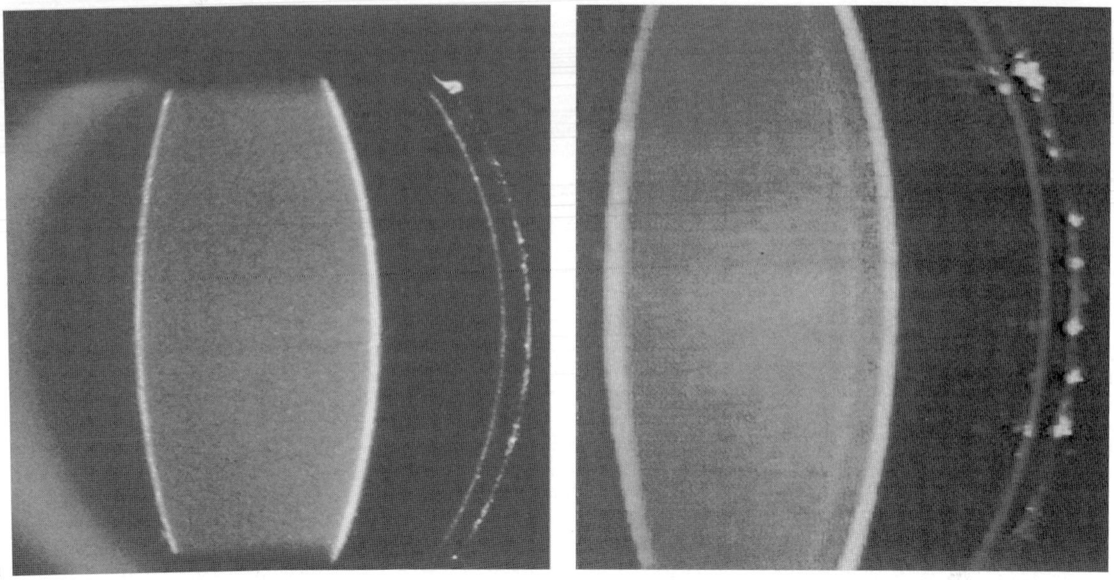

a b

Fig. 7. Images of a phantom eye with flash light. **a** Taken by the photographic unit. **b** Taken by the video unit.

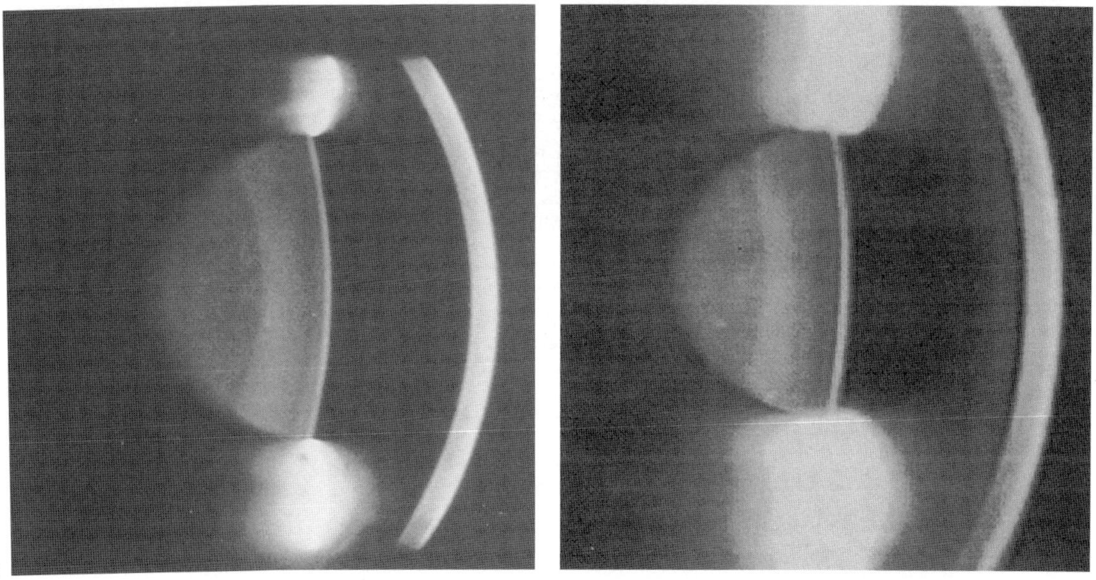

a b

Fig. 8. Anterior eye segment without dilation of the iris and with flash light of a human volunteer (30 years old). **a** Taken by the photographic unit. **b** Taken by the video unit.

clinical and experimental lens and eye research has become available. This SL 45 photo/video system combines the advantages of the other instruments on the market and avoids the great disadvantages of the available on-line instruments with respect to color imaging and fluorescence measurements of the anterior eye segment, mainly the lens.

As far as our experience has shown, reconstruction of the TOPCON SL 45 cameras distributed worldwide will be possible.[4]

---

[4] For information please contact: Mr. Viorel Dragomirescu, Wiesenstrasse 3, D–53424 Remagen-Unkelbach (Germany) Tel. & Fax: xx49–2642–21189.

References

1 Dragomirescu V, Hockwin O, Koch H-R, Sasaki K: Development of a new equipment for rotating slit image photography according to Scheimpflug's principle. Interdiscipl Top Gerontol 1978;13:118–130.

2 Hockwin O, Dragomirescu V, Laser H, Wegener A, Eckerskorn U: Measuring lens transparency by Scheimpflug photography of the anterior eye segment: Principle, instrumentation and application to clinical and experimental ophthalmology. J Toxicol Cut Ocular Toxicol 1987;6:251–271.

3 Hockwin O, Sasaki K, Lerman S: Evaluating cataract development with the Scheimpflug camera; in Masters BR (ed): Noninvasive Diagnostic Techniques in Ophthalmology. Berlin, Springer, 1990, pp 281–318.

4 Hockwin O: Densitometrie der Linse; in Straub W, Kroll P, Küchle HJ (eds): Augenärztliche Untersuchungsmethoden, Aufl. 2. Stuttgart, Enke, 1995, pp 86–106.

5 Niesel P, Müller D: Quantifizierung der senilen Katarakt im Spaltbild des Zeiss SLC-Messsystems. Klin Monatsbl Augenheilk 1988;192: 173–175.

6 Harris ML, Smith GTH, Brown NAP: Inter- and intra-observer reproducibility of the new Oxford CCD Scheimpflug camera. Eye 1991;5:487–490.

7 Sasaki K, Sakamoto Y, Shibata T, Emori Y: The multi-purpose camera: A new anterior eye segment analysis system. Ophthalmic Res 1990;22(suppl 1):3–8.

8 Wegener A, Hockwin O, Laser H, Strack C: Comparison of the Nidek EAS 1000 system and the Topcon SL 45 in clinical application. Ophthalmic Res 1992;24(suppl 1):55–62.

9 Huebscher H-J, Schmidt H: On-line Scheimpflug imaging and its potential for in vivo examination of cornea and lens. Ophthalmic Res 1994; 26(suppl 1):33–38.

10 Egner P, Roos H, Kellerer AM: Applicability and technical features of an electronic Scheimpflug system for cataract studies (abstract). Int Forum on Advanced Techniques in Lens and Cataract Res, Kanazawa, 1995, p 40.

11 Sasaki K, Hiiragi M, Sakamoto Y: Documentation of coloration of crystalline lens in vivo. Jpn J Clin Ophthalmol 1983;37:832–833.

12 Shibata T: In vivo measurement of crystalline lens coloration: Aging changes in non-cataractous eyes and color changes in diabetics. Folia Ophthalmol Jpn 1988:598–605.

13 Lerman S, Hockwin O: UV-visible slit lamp densitography of the human eye. Exp Eye Res 1981;33:587–596.

Ophthalmic Research

Ophthalmic Res 1996;28(suppl 2):109–114

T.R. Shearer
D.B. Throneburg
M. Shih

Departments of Oral Molecular Biology and Ophthalmology, Oregon Health Sciences University, Portland, Oreg., USA

In vitro Precipitation of Rat Lens Crystallins by Calpain I – A Calpain Requiring Low Amounts of Calcium for Activation

Key Words
Crystallins
Calpain I
Precipitation
Rat
Lens
mRNA

Abstract
The overall goal of this study was to provide data on the function and physiologic significance of lens calpain I, a cysteine protease requiring low amounts of calcium for activation. Reverse-transcriptase polymerase chain reaction was used to detect mRNAs for calpains I and II in young rat lenses. An in vitro model of crystallin precipitation was used to assess the ability of calpain I to induce hydrolysis and precipitation of crystallins. We found that incubation of crystallins with purified calpain I was indeed a powerful inducer of crystallin precipitation. However, mRNA levels for calpain I in whole lens appeared to be lower compared to calpain-II mRNA. Participation of calpain I in crystallin precipitation during normal maturation of rodent lenses or cataract formation is thus theoretically possible, but unlikely, because of the low level of expression of calpain I.

Introduction

Calpains (EC 3.4.22.17) are nonlysosomal, calcium-activated, neutral proteases found in almost all tissues studied including lens [1]. Two ubiquitous isoforms of calpain exist in varying proportions in tissues. Although calpain-II enzyme activity is much greater than calpain I in lens [2], calpain I is of interest because of its relatively low calcium requirement. Calpain I (μ-calpain) from lens requires approximately 4 μ*M* calcium for half-maximal activation [2], while calpain II (m-calpain) requires 200–500 μ*M* calcium [3]. Thus, calpain II has been implicated in a wide variety of rodent cataracts [4] where total calcium levels frequently exceed 1 m*M* [5]. A role for insolubilization of crytallins in rodent cata-

KARGER

E-Mail karger@karger.ch
Fax + 41 61 306 12 34
http://www.karger.ch

© 1996 S. Karger AG, Basel

T.R. Shearer
Departments of Oral Molecular Biology and Ophthalmology
Oregon Health Sciences University
611 SW Campus Drive
Portland, OR 97201 (USA)

Table 1. Primer set for PCR for calpains I and II

Target	Upstream primer (5′→3′)	Downstream primer (5′→3′)	Expected PCR product, base pairs
Calpain II (catalytic subunit)	GGG CAG ACC AAC ATC CAC CTC AGC AAA AAC	GTC TCG ATG CTG AAG CCA TCT GAC TTG AT	404
Calpain I (catalytic subunit)	CAC TTG AAG CGT GAC TTC TTC CTG GCC AAT GC	GCA CTC ATG CTG CCC GAC TTG TCC AGG TCA AAC TT	536

racts after proteolysis by calpain II was supported by a recent in vitro model. In this model, crystallins from young rat lens were partially hydrolyzed and precipitated when incubated with purified calpain II [6] or by activation of endogenous lens calpain [7]. No information is available as to whether or not calpain I can cause similar precipitation. Therefore, one purpose of this report was to determine whether calpain I can induce precipitation of crystallins in vitro. The other purpose was to measure mRNA levels for calpain I and II in lens in order to assess their relative physiologic importance.

Materials and Methods

Precipitation of Crystallins with Purified Calpain I in vitro

Experimental animals were handled in compliance with the 'Guiding Principles in Care and Use of Animals' (DHEW Publication, NIH 86-23). Lenses with capsular epithelium were obtained by a posterior approach from 12-day-old Sprague-Dawley rats (B & K International) after CO_2 inhalation. Twenty lenses were homogenized per milliliter of buffer I containing 20 m*M* imidazole (pH 7.0), 50 μ*M* EGTA, 0.02% NaN_3, and 2 m*M* fresh dithioerythritol. Soluble proteins were obtained by centrifugation at 16,000 *g* for 5 min and assayed for protein using the Bio-Rad dye-binding reagent with BSA as standard.

For light-scattering measurements [7], each well of half-well, flat-bottom, microtiter plates (Costar Corp., Cambridge, Mass., USA; catalog No. 3690) contained in a total volume of 80 μl buffer I (final concentrations): 20 mg/ml rat lens soluble proteins, 12 μg purified calpain I from porcine erythrocytes (Nacalai Tesque, Kyoto, Japan) per mg protein, and 1,600 μ*M* Ca^{2+} to initiate the experiment and activate calpain. Negative controls were identical, except they contained 100 μ*M* E64 (Peptide Institute, Japan) to inhibit calpain. The microtiter plates were covered with pressure-sensitive tape (Costar, No. 3095) and incubated at 36 °C. Light-scattering in each well was determined in an ELISA microtiter plate reader (Anthos LabTech Instruments, Salzburg, Austria; model HtII) by measuring absorbance at 405 nm. Light-scattering in wells from each treatment group was averaged, and values are reported as change in mOD units ($\Delta OD \times 1{,}000$) after subtracting the initial light-scattering of lens soluble proteins at time O.

For SDS-PAGE, 5–6 μg protein were loaded per lane onto pre-cast, 1.5-mm-thick, 8 × 8 cm, 18% polyacrylamide mini-gels (Novex, San Diego, Calif., USA, catalog No. EC6508). Proteins were separated using the Tris-glycine buffer system in a Novex Xcell-II chamber [8]. Proteins were stained with Coomassie Brilliant blue R-250.

Detection of mRNAs for Calpains I and II by Polymerase Chain Reaction

Lenses from rats were sonicated in guanidine isothiocyanate, and RNA was then isolated by the Glass-MAX RNA microisolation spin cartridge system (Gibco BRL, catalog No. 8385SA) and treated with DNAse to remove genomic DNA. Total RNA was subsequently converted to single-stranded cDNA with reverse transcriptase (RT) and the appropriate gene-specific downstream primer (table 1), based on the known sequences of rat calpain I [Dr. John Elce, Queens University, pers. commun.] and calpain II [9]. The cDNA was treated with RNAse (Gibco BRL SuperScript

PreAmplification System (Catalog No. 18089-011). Polymerase chain reaction (PCR) in 50 μl reaction mixtures was then performed on cDNA by adding the appropriate gene-specific primers (table 1). PCR conditions optimized for calpain I were: initial denaturation at 95 °C for 4 min, and then 35 cycles were performed on a PTC-100 thermal cycler (MJ Research Inc., Watertown, Mass., USA) at denaturation, 94 °C for 45 s; primer annealing, 66 °C for 45 s; primer extension 72 °C for 60 s, and final primer extension, 72 °C for 10 min. Optimized conditions for calpain II were: initial denaturation at 94 °C for 2 min, and then 35 cycles at denaturation, 94 °C for 45 s; primer annealing, 55 °C for 45 s; primer extension 72 °C for 60 s, and final primer extension, 72 °C for 10 min. PCR products were visualized on 1.5% ethidium-bromide-stained gels, and Polaroid pictures (type 667) were scanned and digitized with a flatbed scanner (Apple Color One). NIH Image software (version 1.57, obtained through Internet via anonymous ftp from zippy.nimh.nih.gov) was used to invert the image to give more easily read dark bands on a white background (fig. 2).

Results

Purified calpain I caused a rapid increase in light-scattering in the total soluble proteins from lens of 12-day-old rats within 20 min after activation with 1.6 m*M* calcium (fig. 1). The E64 control group (fig. 1) was incubated under the same conditions except for the addition of 106 μ*M* E64, which is an inhibitor of cysteine proteases such as calpain [10]. The E64 group showed very little light-scattering. This indicated that the large increase in light-scattering in the calpain-I group was due to the action of calpain and not due to direct precipitation of crystallins by calcium. Note that the addition of calcium also undoubtedly activated endogenous calpain II causing proteolysis of α- and β-crystallins [7]. However, precipitation of crystallins by endogenous calpain II is not appreciable until after several days (data not shown).

The pattern of proteolysis from incubation with calpain I observed by SDS-PAGE (fig. 1, insert) was similar to the pattern produced by purified calpain II [6]. This included loss of βB1 and accumulation of lower-molecular-weight fragments below α-crystallin. This indicated that calpain I does not produce additional fragments that appear grossly different in size than from calpain II.

The data above suggest that both calpains I and II are able to induce similar proteolysis and precipitation of crystallins from lenses of young rats. Previous studies indicated that enzymatic activity in lens, and total amount of calpain-II protein (immunoreactivity) are much higher than for calpain I [2, 11, 12]. However, we did not know whether this was due to low transcription of mRNA for calpain I. mRNAs for calpains were assessed qualitatively with RT-PCR in the present experiment using gene-specific primers for calpains I and II (fig. 2, upper gel). Rat lens cDNA yielded PCR products at the correctly predicted sizes of 536 and 404 bp for calpains I and II, respectively. Although PCR conditions were separately optimized for both calpains I and II, the data are only qualitative since they were not corrected for potential differences in amplifying efficiencies of the primers for calpains I and II. The band for calpain I was present but fainter, and thus the amount of mRNA for calpain I appeared to be less than for calpain II. The same conclusion was reached using oligo (dT) primer in the initial RT reaction, and mRNA for calpain I was also lower than for calpain II in murine lenses (data not shown). For comparison purposes, mRNAs for calpains I and II were also visualized in other tissues from young rats (fig. 2, lower gel). Brain and lung seemed to have abundant amounts of calpain-I mRNA. Quantitative RT-PCR showed that amounts of calpain-II mRNA in young rat lenses were 3–5 times higher than in these other tissues [Ma and Shearer, unpubl. results].

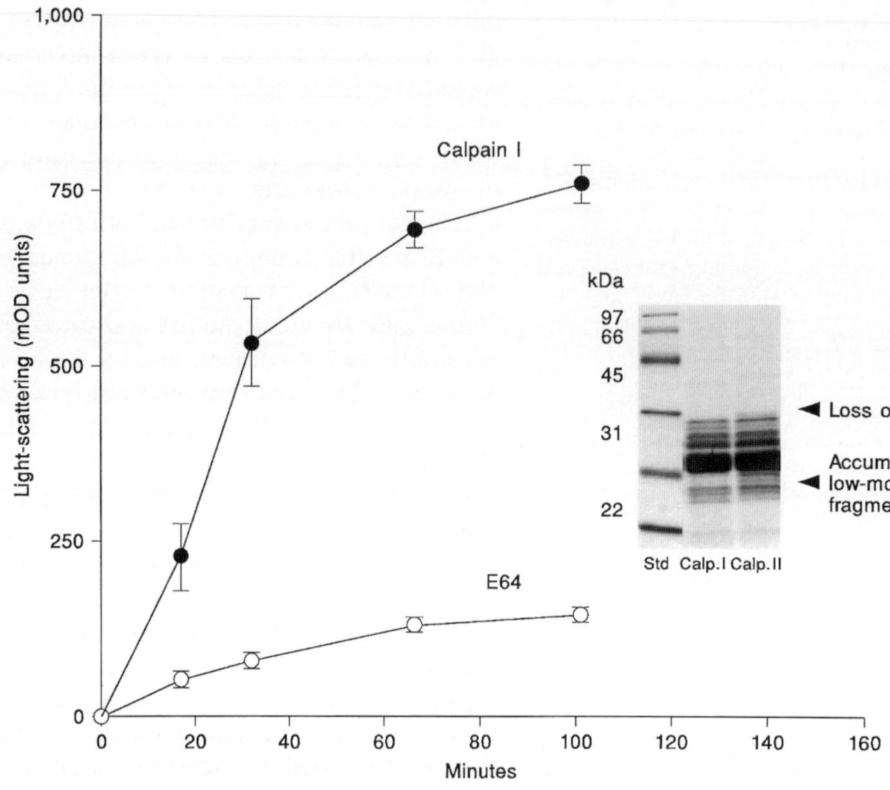

Fig. 1. Light-scattering in the total soluble proteins from young rat lens during incubation with calpain I (upper curve) or with E64 protease inhibitor (lower curve). Minutes on x-axis indicate the time after addition of 1.6 m*M* calcium to both groups containing 12 μg calpain-I/mg protein and 20 mg total soluble proteins/ml. Y-axis is light-scattering at A_{405} expressed as OD units × 10^3 = mOD. In this experiment, bars at the mean data points represent standard deviation for 5 replicate wells for the calpain-I group and 3 replicate wells for the E64 control group. **Insert.** SDS-PAGE of rat lens proteins in incubation wells of a separate experiment after treatment with calcium and purified calpains I (lane 2) or II (lane 3). The first lane (Std) contains molecular-weight marker proteins with masses in kilodaltons on the left. Note the similar pattern of proteolysis in lanes 2 and 3 with either isoform of calpain. A complete description of changes in SDS-PAGE after incubation with calpain II compared to control has been published elsewhere [6].

Discussion

The data above demonstrated mRNAs for both calpains I and II in rat lens. Previous studies have found mRNAs for calpain I and II in other tissues or cell types [13], but, to our knowledge, these are the only comparative data on the 2 mRNAs in lens. Our data appeared to show relatively lower amounts of calpain-I mRNA in lens compared to calpain II. This helps to explain the low levels of calpain-I enzyme activity in lens. However, be-

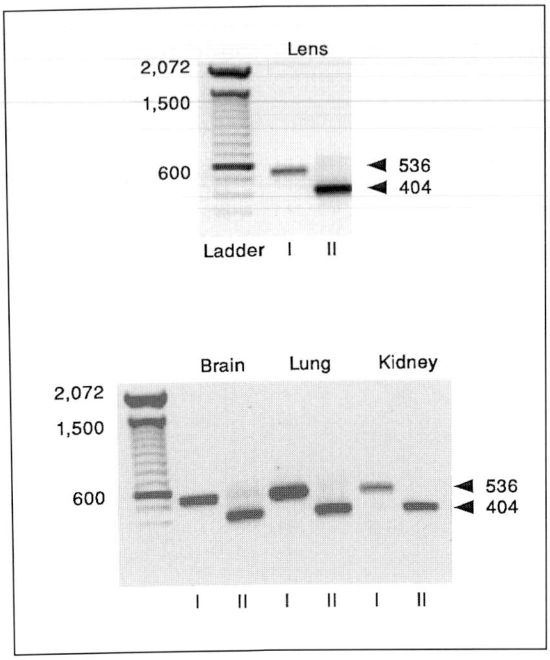

Fig. 2. RT-PCR analysis of mRNAs for calpains I and II in lens (upper gel) and other tissues (lower) from lens of young rats visualized on an ethidium-bromide-stained agarose gel. Lane 1 contains a 100-bp ladder; the 600-, 1,500- and 2,072-bp bands are marked and are brighter than others. The top arrow indicates the migration position of PCR products from calpain-I cDNA at the predicted 536-bp position, while the lower arrow shows a band for calpain II at 404 bp. Each lane represents 100 ng total RNA.

sides not correcting for PCR-amplifying efficiencies in our PCR reactions, the RNA utilized in the present study was isolated from whole lens; while calpain-I enzyme activity was found to be concentrated in the capsule epithelium of bovine lens [2]. Using quantitative RT-PCR, we recently found mRNAs for calpain II to be 3 times higher in the capsular-epithelium-cortex preparations than in nucleus [Hong and Shearer, unpubl. observ.]. The present studies may thus be underestimating calpain-I and -II mRNA levels in the more metabolically active regions of the lens. An immunohistologic study or in situ hybridization description of the regional distribution of calpains in lens is needed to more fully understand the site of action of calpains. However, low levels of expression or enzymatic activity do not necessarily mean that the enzyme has no important function. For example, the mRNA for tissue-specific calpain, p94, was found exclusively in skeletal muscle, yet protein levels were not detected [14], which suggested that this calpain is rapidly degraded after performing a specific function. mRNAs for two other tissue-specific calpains, nCL-2 and nCL-2′, are found predominantly in the stomach. A search for lens-specific calpains would be interesting since such data would help determine whether they or the ubiquitous calpains I and II are important in lens biochemistry.

The data above are the first to demonstrate that purified calpain I was able to precipitate crystallins from young rat lens in vitro. The time course and pattern of proteolysis were similar to the well-characterized in vitro precipitation of crystallins by calpain II [6]. Cleavage sites on the insoluble β-crystallin fragments after incubation with calpain II were also similar to calpain-like cleavage sites found on β-crystallin fragments in selenite cataracts [15]. These data suggest a common mechanism for crystallin precipitation with calpains I and II. We hypothesize that the loss of N-termini on β-crystallins leads to exposure of hydrophobic regions and precipitation. Because of the much larger amounts of calpain II and the massive increase in lens calcium, a role for calpain I in the precipitation of lens crystallins during cataract formation in rodents is doubtful. However, during lens maturation, calpain I may be preferentially activated by transient, localized spikes of calcium not high enough to activate calpain II. Numerous β-crystallin fragments containing calpain-like cleavage sites have been found in the insoluble protein formed during normal maturation of rat lens nucleus [16], which indicated that some form of calpain is activated under the low-calcium conditions in maturing lens. The data in the present investigation showed that calpain I could theoretically participate in production of insoluble fragments found in normal rodent lenses. However, because of the lower level of expression, such a mechanism seems unlikely unless calpain I is subsequently found to be concentrated in some specific region of lens.

Acknowledgments

Supported by NEI grant No. EY03600 and EY05786 to T.R.S. The authors wish to thank Drs. Hong Ma and Larry David for helpful discussions.

References

1 Corall DE, DeMartino GN: Calcium-activated neutral protease (calpain) system: Structure, function and regulation. Physiol Rev 1991; 71:813–847.

2 Yoshida H, Murachi T, Tsukahara I: Distribution of calpain I, calpain II and calpastatin in bovine lens. Invest Ophthalmol Vis Sci 1985;26: 953–956.

3 David LL, Shearer TR: Purification of calpain II from rat lens and determination of endogenous substrates. Exp Eye Res 1986;42:227–238.

4 Kadoya K, Azuma M, David LL, Shearer TR: Role of calpain in hydrogen peroxide induced cataract. Curr Eye Res 1993;12:341–346.

5 Shearer TR, David LL: Role of calcium in selenium cataract. Curr Eye Res 1983;2:777–784.

6 David LL, Wright JW, Shearer TR: Calpain II induced insolubilization of lens β-crystallin polypeptides may induce cataract. Biochim Biophys Acta 1992;1139:210–216.

7 Shearer TR, Shih M, Azuma A, David LL: Precipitation of crystallins from young rat lens by endogenous calpain. Exp Eye Res 1995;61: 141–150.

8 Laemmli UK: Cleavage of structural proteins during assembly of head of bacteriophage. Nature 1970;227: 680–685.

9 DeLuca CI, Davies PL, Samis JA, Elce J: Molecular cloning and bacterial expression of cDNA for rat calpain II 80 Da subunit. Biochim Acta 1993;1216:81–93.

10 Azuma M, David LL, Shearer TR: superior prevention of calcium ionophore cataract by E64d. Biochim Biophys Acta 1992;1180:215–220.

11 Varnum MD, David LL, Shearer TR: Age-related changes in calpain II and calpastatin in rat lens. Exp Eye Res 1989;49:1053–1065.

12 David LL, Varnum MD, Lampi KJ, Shearer TR: Calpain II in human lenses. Invest Ophthalmol Vis Sci 1989;30:269–275.

13 Poussard S, Cottin P, Brustis JJ, Talmat S, Elamrani N, Ducostaing A: Quantitative measurement of calpain I and II mRNAs in differentiating rat muscle cells using competitive polymerase chain reaction method. Biochimie 1993;75:885–890.

14 Saido TC, Sorimachi H, Susuki K: Calpain: New perspectives in molecular diversity and physiological-pathological involvement. FASEB J 1994;8:814–822.

15 David LL, Shearer TR: β-Crystallins insolubilized by calpain II in vitro contain cleavage sites similar to β-crystallins insolubilized during cataract. FEBS Lett 1993;324:265–270.

16 David LL, Azuma M, Shearer TR: Cataract and the acceleration of calpain-induced β-crystallin insolubilization occurring during normal maturation of rat lens. Invest Ophthalmol Vis Sci 1994;35:785–793.

Ophthalmic Research

Ophthalmic Res 1996;28(suppl 2):115–119

Barry R. Masters

Department of Anatomy and Cell Biology, Uniformed Services University of the Health Sciences, Bethesda, Md., USA

Three-Dimensional Confocal Microscopy of the Lens

Key Words
Confocal microscopy
Three-dimensional imaging
Lens epithelium
Lens suture
Lens fibers

Abstract
A confocal microscopic technique is described to obtain optical sections from the in situ ocular lens of the rabbit and mouse. Optical sections were obtained with blue light through the full thickness of the lens epithelium, and of the anterior lenticular fibers. An image showing the structure of an anterior suture was obtained from the murine lens. A three-dimensional volume visualization of lenticular fibers from the anterior region of the rabbit lens was reconstructed from a stack of optical sections. These in situ microscopic observations of unstained, unfixed specimens correspond to previous studies using electron microscopy.

Introduction

Optical microscopy of the lens could, with further development, permit observation of dynamical changes of structure and morphology. There is a need to observe the lens in unstained, unfixed, living specimens. For example, the in vivo observation of cell growth, migration, differentiation and alterations of lens epithelium, lenticular fibers, and the capsule would be useful in animal models of cataract and drug ocular toxicity.

A real-time laser scan confocal microscope (LSCM) has been developed for the in vivo human eye with the capability to image the lens suture and posterior capsule [1]. However, further technical improvements are necessary before it can image the fine structure of lens epithelium and lenticular fibers.

Before general clinical use of in vivo confocal microscopy it is first necessary to establish a correlation between optical microscopy and electron microscopy. The three-dimensional organization of lens fibers in the rabbit was investigated with scanning electron microsco-

KARGER

E-Mail karger@karger.ch
Fax + 41 61 306 12 34
http://www.karger.ch

© 1996 S. Karger AG, Basel

Prof. Barry R. Masters
Department of Anatomy and Cell Biology
Uniformed Services University of the Health Sciences
4301 Jones Bridge Road
Bethesda, MD 20814-4799 (USA)

py [2]. The structure of the in situ rabbit lens was studied with a LSCM [3]. Recent improvements in specimen preparation have improved our ability to obtain optical sections from an in situ lens of an ex vivo rabbit eye [4].

This study demonstrates the use of confocal microscopy to study unfixed, unstained ocular lens. It revealed the fine structure of lens epithelium, anterior suture, anterior lenticular fibers, and the three-dimensional arrangement of lens fibers.

Materials and Methods

Sources of Material

Eyes were obtained from male New Zealand white rabbits weighing 2.5–3.0 kg and from Balb-c mice. The animals were maintained and handled in accordance with the 'Resolution on the Use of Animals in Research', of the Association for Research in Vision and Ophthalmology (Bethesda, Md., USA). The rabbits were anesthetized with an intramuscular injection of ketamine HCl (40 mg/kg) and xylazine (5 mg/kg). Mice were killed by cervical dislocation and the proptosed eye was cut off at the optic nerve. The eyes were freed of adhering tissue and swiftly removed. They were immediately placed in a beaker containing bicarbonate Ringer's solution with glucose (5 m*M*) and calcium (2 m*M*) at 25 °C.

Confocal Microscopy

Image Acquisition. The lenses were observed in situ with a BioRad© MRC-600 LSCM. The microscope was operated in the back-scattered-light mode. The laser excitation was a 25-mW argon ion laser with excitation lines at 488 and 514 nm.

Each optical section was acquired as a compilation of 10 separate scanned frames averaged using the Kalman algorithm. The lens was then scanned moving the stage of the microscope exactly 1 μm in the z-axis between frames, thus producing a data set whose individual pixels represent isometrically cubic voxels.

The LSCM detector aperture was opened to one quarter full size. The light detector was a photomultiplier (Thorn EMI 9828B) with an S-20 photocathode. The photomultiplier output was digitized to 8 bits, which resulted in images with a dynamic range of 256 gray levels.

A Nikon Optiphot microscope with a ×10 ocular was coupled to the LSCM. The microscope objective was a Leitz ×25 water immersion objective with numerical aperture of 0.6, with a free working distance of 1.7 mm. The eyes were placed in a container that gently provided mechanical stability and minimized the mechanical motion of the eye [4].

Three-Dimensional Volume Reconstructions. The stacks of two-dimensional optical sections were collected by computer control of the Nikon Optiphot microscope equipped with a stepping motor. The data sets were transferred to a Silicon Graphics Personal IRIS 4D/35G via an Ethernet connection. The data sets were all converted into a readable format by running an extract program to remove the BioRad header files. The data sets were reconstructed using Voxel View Software (Vital Images, Fairfield, Iowa, USA).

Results

Confocal microscopy of the lens was performed from an in situ lens in an ex vivo rabbit eye. Optical sections were obtained from the anterior of the lens epithelium through the lenticular fibers in the anterior of the lens. The lens epithelium and its relation to the lens fibers is shown in figure 1a. The plane of focus of the confocal microscope was moved from the surface of the lens epithelium, to the junction of the epithelium and the fibers and finally into the anterior fibers. The cell borders of epithelial cells showed bright reflections and high contrast. The optical section included both the posterior region of the epithelial cells and the anterior region of the lens fibers as shown in figure 1b. The smaller-diameter lens from the mouse was used to demonstrate the structure of the anterior suture. A typical region of the anterior suture of the murine lens in situ is shown in figure 2. The suture region appears to scatter more light than the nonsuture region of the lens.

Confocal microscopy of the in situ rabbit lens shows the typical optical section of the lens fibers in the anterior region of the lens. An optical section focused on an array of par-

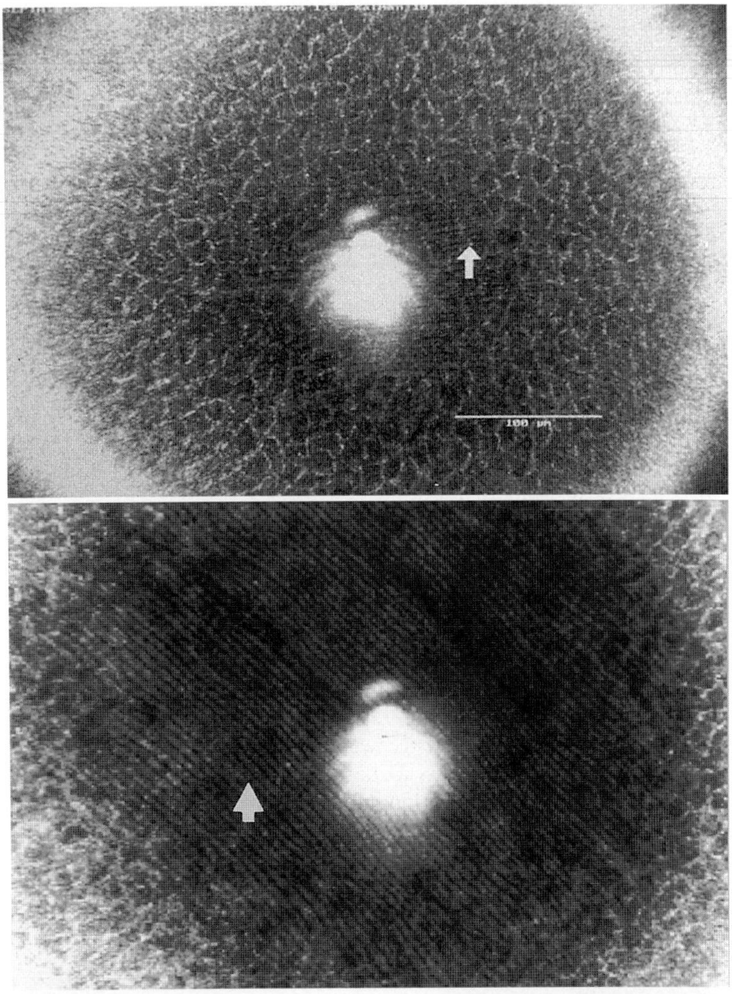

a

b

Fig. 1. Confocal microscopic image of in situ rabbit lens. **a** Optical section of posterior lens epithelial cells and anterior lenticular fibers (arrow). Scale bar = 100 µm. **b** Optical section showing surface lenticular fibers and lens epithelial cells in periphery of image.

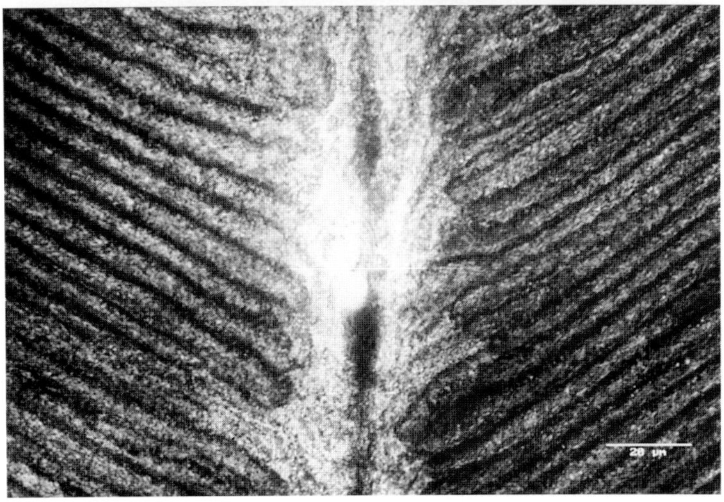

Fig. 2. Confocal microscopic image of anterior suture of an ex vivo murine lens. Scale bar = 20 µm.

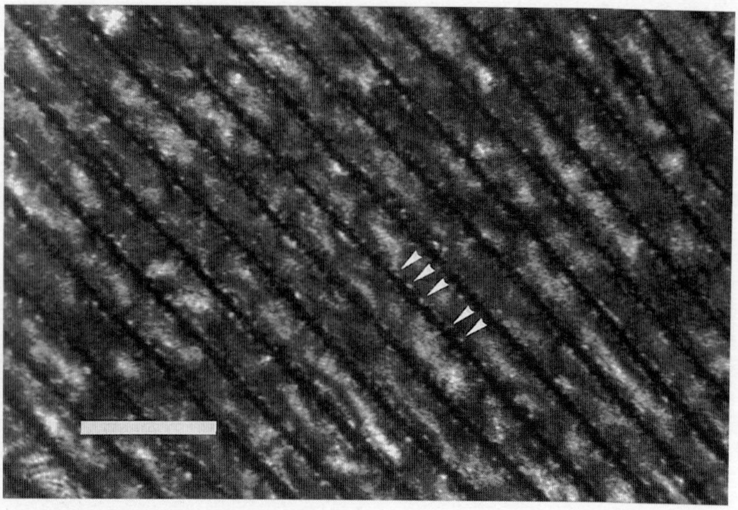

Fig. 3. Confocal microscopic image of lenticular fibers of in situ rabbit lens located 100 μm posterior to the lens epithelium under the anterior pole. The repeat distance in the optical section is 7 μm. Arrowheads indicate bright spots on fiber edges. Scale bar = 20 μm.

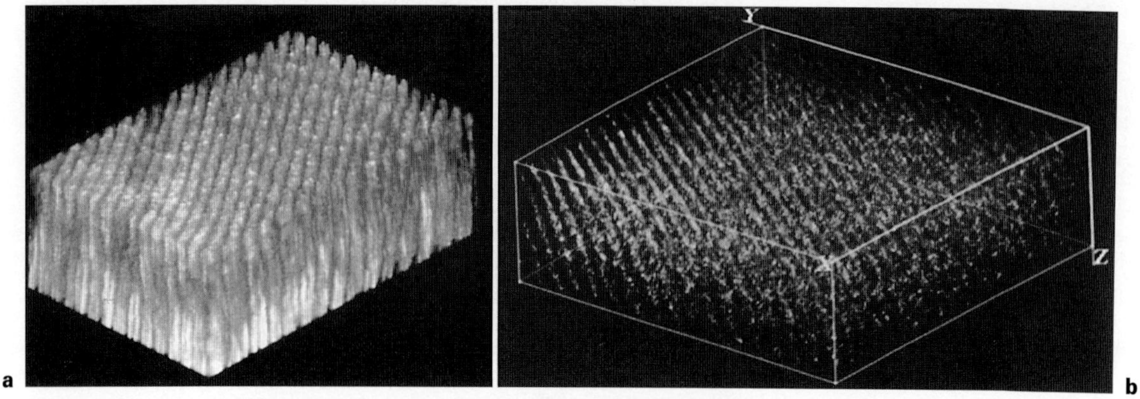

Fig. 4. Three-dimensional volume visualization of in situ rabbit lens. **a** Visualization of oblique section aligned parallel to fibers showing orientation of lenticular fibers under anterior pole of lens. **b** Visualization of oblique section slightly rotated from previous view and reconstructed with increased transparency.

allel fibers is shown in figure 3. Variations in reflectivity from various regions of the fibers are observed. At the edges of the fibers arrays of bright dots were observed.

A three-dimensional visualization of a volume of the anterior lens from the in situ rabbit lens is shown in figure 4a. This figure demonstrates the alignment and orientation of lenticular fibers from the anterior lens. A three-dimensional visualization with a slightly different orientation and increased transparency is shown in figure 4b.

Discussion

These studies of the in situ lens in an ex vivo eye demonstrate that there is sufficient inherent contrast in the ocular lens when observed with confocal microscopy. This encouraging result means that further advances in confocal microscopy of the in vivo lens should result in images of similar contrast. The fine structure of the lens epithelium, lens suture, and lenticular fibers correlate with studies of fixed material using scanning electron microscopy.

The cell borders of lens epithelial cells are observed across the full thickness of the lens epithelium. The series of bright spots along the edges of lenticular fibers may be interlocking protrusions of lens fibers in the rabbit under electron-microscopic investigations [2].

This study demonstrates the ability of confocal microscopy to obtain optical sections of the full thickness of the lens epithelium. This capability could be important in animal toxicity studies of material that effects the integrity of the epithelial cells. The ability to form three-dimensional visualizations of the anterior lenticular fibers may be useful to follow alterations of lenticular morphology in the anterior surface of the lens.

The use of confocal microscopy to study the in situ ocular lens currently has several limitations. The bow region of the lens where lens epithelial cells differentiate into lens fibers may not be readily observed due to the iris. The ability to image the full thickness of the lens will require a new design with a free working distance that can reach about 1 cm from the anterior surface of the cornea to the posterior surface of the lens. There is also the problem of light penetration into the lens and the limited amount of light that is scattered back into the collection optics of the imaging system. It is suggested that longer wavelengths of light may be more suitable for deeper penetration of highly scattering ocular tissue.

Acknowledgment

This work was supported by a grant from NIH EY-06958.

References

1 Massig JH, Preissler M, Wegener AR, Gaida G: Real-time confocal laser scan microscope for examination and diagnosis of the eye in vivo. Appl Optics 1994;33:690–694.

2 Willekens B, Vrensen G: The three-dimensional organization of lens fibers in the rabbit. Albrecht von Graefes Arch Klin Exp Ophthalmol 1981;216:275–289.

3 Masters BR: Confocal microscopy of the in-situ crystalline lens. J Microsc 1991;165:159–167.

4 Masters BR: Specimen preparation and chamber for confocal microscopy of the ex vivo eye. Scanning Microsc 1993;7:645–651.

Ophthalmic Research

Ophthalmic Res 1996;28(suppl 2):120–126

Three-Dimensional Volume Visualization of the in vivo Human Ocular Lens Showing Localization of the Cataract

Barry R. Masters [b]
Kazuyuki Sasaki [a]
Yasuo Sakamoto [a]
Masami Kojima [a]
Yasufumi Emori [a]
Stephen L. Senft [c]
Murray Foster [d]

[a] Department of Ophthalmology, Kanazawa Medical University, Uchinada-Macchi, Ishikawa-Ken, Japan;
[b] Department of Anatomy and Cell Biology, Uniformed Services University of the Health Sciences, Bethesda, Md., and
[c] Department of Psychology, Yale University, and Neuroengineering and Neuroscience Center, New Haven, Conn., and
[d] Vital Images, Inc., Fairfield, Iowa, USA

Key Words
Three-dimensional lens imaging
Cataract
Three-dimensional volume-rendering

Abstract

An in vivo human lens containing a cataract has been visualized by volume rendering a transformed series of 60 rotated Scheimpflug digital images. The data set was obtained by rotating the Scheimpflug camera about the optic axis of the lens in 3-degree increments. The set of 60 Scheimpflug digital images were mathematically transformed into a new data set in which the images are oriented perpendicular to the optic axis of the eye. The transformed set of optical sections were first aligned to correct for eye movements during the data collection process, then rendered into a three-dimensional volume reconstruction with volume-rendering computer graphics techniques. The viewpoint and the transparency of the volume rendered in vivo human lens were varied in order to observe volume opacities in various regions of the lens. To help visualize lens opacities, the intensity of light scattering was pseudocolor-coded as an integral part of the three-dimensional volume rendering. Three-dimensional, pseudocolored volume rendering of the in vivo human ocular lens represents a new technique to visualize in vivo human cataracts.

Introduction

The ability to observe the in vivo human ocular lens is an important factor in lens and cataract research. It is possible to image regions of the in vivo lens with different optical instruments. The lens epithelium was observed in vivo by specular illumination at the slit lamp microscope [1, 2]. A specular microscope was used to image in vivo human lenses [3, 4].

KARGER

E-Mail karger@karger.ch
Fax + 41 61 306 12 34
http://www.karger.ch

© 1996 S. Karger AG, Basel

Prof. Barry R. Masters
Department of Anatomy and Cell Biology
Uniformed Services University of the
Health Sciences, 4301 Jones Bridge Road
Bethesda, MD 20814-4799 (USA)

The development of the Scheimpflug camera has enabled the ophthalmologist to obtain sharp, two-dimensional images of sections across the full thickness of the ocular lens [5, 6].

In recent years there have been several developments in three-dimensional visualization of ocular tissues. Volume-rendering methods were used for the first three-dimensional reconstruction of the full thickness of an ex vivo rabbit cornea [7]. Subsequent studies by Masters and Farmer [8] developed the three-dimensional visualization of the cornea and the lens in an intact ex vivo rabbit eye. These techniques were also extended to the in vivo human retina [9].

Our choice of volume-rendering computer techniques to generate a three-dimensional visualization of ocular tissues from a set of two-dimensional slices is based on the following characteristics [10]. Volume rendering does not require a prior specification of surface geometry of the object. Surfaces appear naturally in the rendered volume. Volume-rendering techniques use all of the data points from the set of slices to form the final image in three dimensions. This is important for objects with poorly defined features such as opacities in the human ocular lens.

The methodology of three-dimensional visualization of the in vivo human lens was first developed by Emori et al. [11]. Their previous studies did not use volume-rendering techniques, but implemented a linear interpolation method to generate 150 coronal sections which were combined to form a gray scale three-dimensional reconstruction [11, 12].

Our current study differs from the previous studies in several ways. We use a new interpolation procedure to convert the rotated set of Scheimpflug images into a new aligned orthogonal set of 332 images. A new volume-rendering software program is used for rendering, viewpoint control, and opacity control of the resulting three-dimensional lens. Pseudocolor was mapped onto the reconstructed volume, as an integral part of the volume-rendering process, to aid in the topological visualization of the opacities in the in vivo human lens.

Materials and Methods

Image Acquisition

The subject of this study was a 68-year-old male volunteer with incipient cataract. Informed consent was given for the imaging of the lens. the subject had anterior and posterior cortical opacities judged to be grade I.

The subject's right eye was dilated with 0.5% tropicamide and 0.5% phenylephrine hydrochloride prior to the Scheimpflug imaging. Sixty Scheimpflug images were acquired with the anterior eye segment analysis system (Nidek, EAS-1000). The Scheimpflug camera was rotated about the optic axis of the patient's eye in 3-degree increments [12]. The data acquisition time was 20 min. Each digital image was 640 by 400 pixels. The ditital images had a dynamic range of 8 bits or 256 gray levels.

Alignment

The acquired Scheimpflug images were not in registration due to eye movements during the image acquisition process. The Scheimpflug images were realigned interactively. One image was chosen as the fiduciary, and two landmarks from the iris reflections were identified. All sequential images were aligned to this first image. The alignment consisted of an xy-shift, a rotation, and a scaling.

Image Resampling

Image resampling refers to the procedure for converting the aligned set of 60 rotated Scheimpflug images into a new set of 332 images by a bilinear interpolation method [submitted for publication]. The new resampled set of images is orthogonal to the optic axis, and consists of slices from the anterior pole to the posterior pole of the ocular lens.

Image Reconstruction by Volume-Rendering Technique

This aligned, resampled data set was processed with VoxelView® (Vital Images, Fairfield, Iowa) software to form three-dimensional volume reconstructions of the in vivo human ocular lens. The software is based on the volume-rendering technique [10].

The voxels in the three-dimensional reconstruction were pseudocolored during the volume rendering to aid in visualization of small differences in opacity in the lens. The pseudocolor coding of the intensity of light scattering from the three-dimensional volume reconstruction of the in vivo human lens is as follows. Dark colors (purple, blue, blue-green) represent low-light-scattering voxels (high lens transparency) and bright colors (green, yellow, orange, red) represent high-light-scattering voxels (low lens transparency). Voxels are small volume elements which comprise the digital, three-dimensional volume.

The volume reconstruction of the in vivo human ocular lens is a three-dimensional digital data set. It can be viewed from any perspective and direction. In order to 'look inside' the three-dimensional volume, the transparency of a subset of the voxels forming the lens can be increased. For example, in order to view the opacities in the anterior regions of the ocular lens, we increased the transparency of the voxels that form the lens epithelium. When the volume is rendered under these conditions, with a viewpoint located in front of the ocular lens, we can 'look inside' the lens and see the cataract located posterior to the lens epithelium.

Results

Several images of the three-dimensional volume reconstruction of the in vivo human ocular lens from different perspectives are shown for illustrative purposes. All of the figures show three-dimensional renderings of the in vivo human lens.

The three-dimensional volume renderings are placed within a yellow cubic wire frame to fix the orientation of the rendering in space. When the rendering is seen directly from the front or from the side, the yellow wire frame is seen as a rectangle. Figure 1a shows an oblique view of the three-dimensional ocular lens. The slight opacities are shown just posterior to the lens epithelium. The bright circular ring is a portion of the iris. Figure 1b shows a frontal view of the three-dimensional reconstruction of the ocular lens. The ring of reflections from the iris is colored orange. The yellow, green, brown, and orange voxels of high opacity (cataract) are clearly shown on the lower right quadrant and in the upper right quadrant of the anterior region of the ocular lens. Figure 1c shows an oblique view from the posterior side of the ocular lens. Opacities in the posterior and more anterior regions are shown. Figure 1d shows an isometric posterior view of the lens. The three-dimensional lens shown in figure 1c has been rotated about the vertical axis. Opacities in the anterior and posterior regions are shown. Figure 1e is a view from the side of the three-dimensional reconstruction of the ocular lens. The midcortical regions of opacity are shown as yellow-orange voxels. Towards the posterior region of the lens nucleus there is a large region of opacity. In the lower cortical region there is a small yellow-orange region of opacity. Figure 1f shows a side view of the three-dimensional reconstruction of the ocular lens. The

(For figures 1c–1f see pages 124/125.)

Fig. 1. A series of three-dimensional volume renderings of the in vivo human lens as viewed from different directions. The yellow box helps to visualize the three-dimensional lens. The bright circular reflection is from the iris. **a** Oblique frontal view shows the lens from the lens epithelium to the posterior lens volume. **b** Frontal view shows anterior regions which contain specific local regions of opacity. **c** Oblique view from the posterior side of the ocular lens. Opacities in the posterior regions and in more anterior regions are shown. **d** An isometric posterior view showing the lens. The three-dimensional lens shown in **c** has been rotated about the vertical axis. Opacities in the anterior and posterior regions are shown. **e** Side view of the full volume of the lens. The anterior and posterior curvature of the in vivo lens is shown. A portion of the highly light-scattering iris is shown as well as anterior and posterior regions of opacity. **f** This view is similar to that shown in **e**; however the three-dimensional lens is rotated about the optic axis by 45°, and is shown with increased transparency.

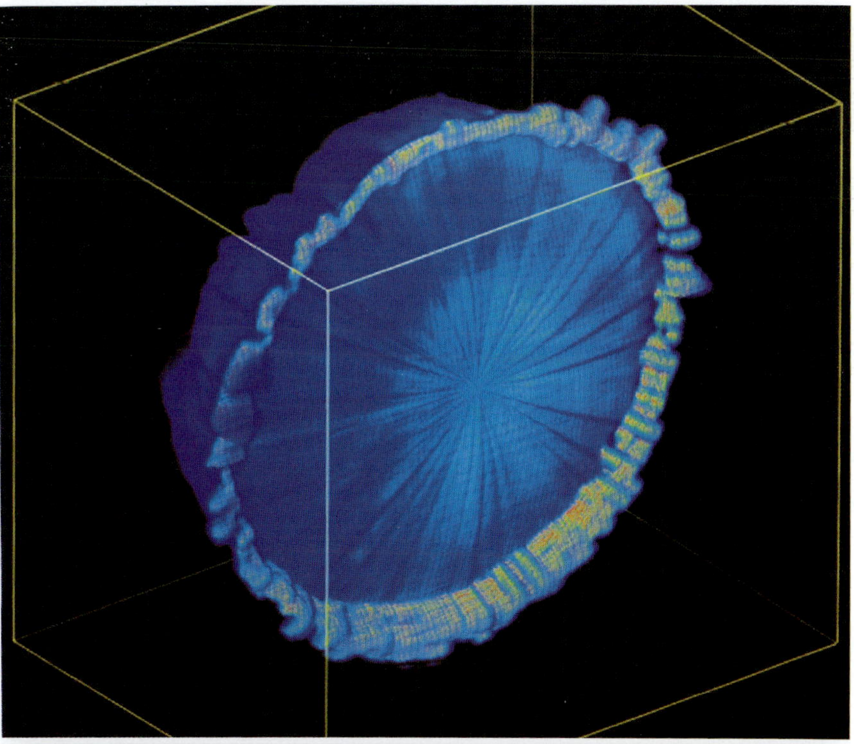

1a

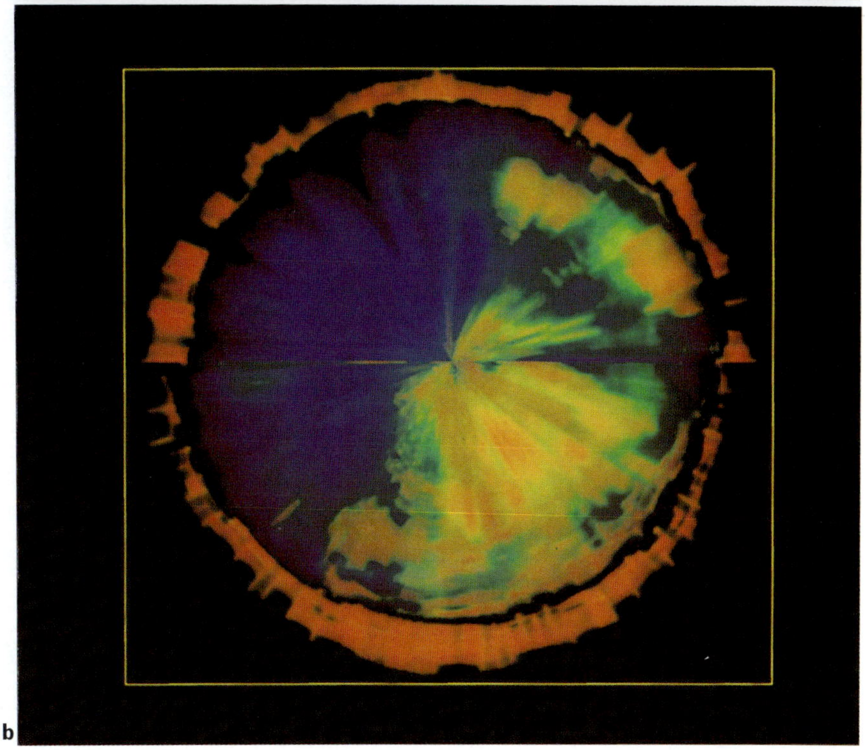

1b

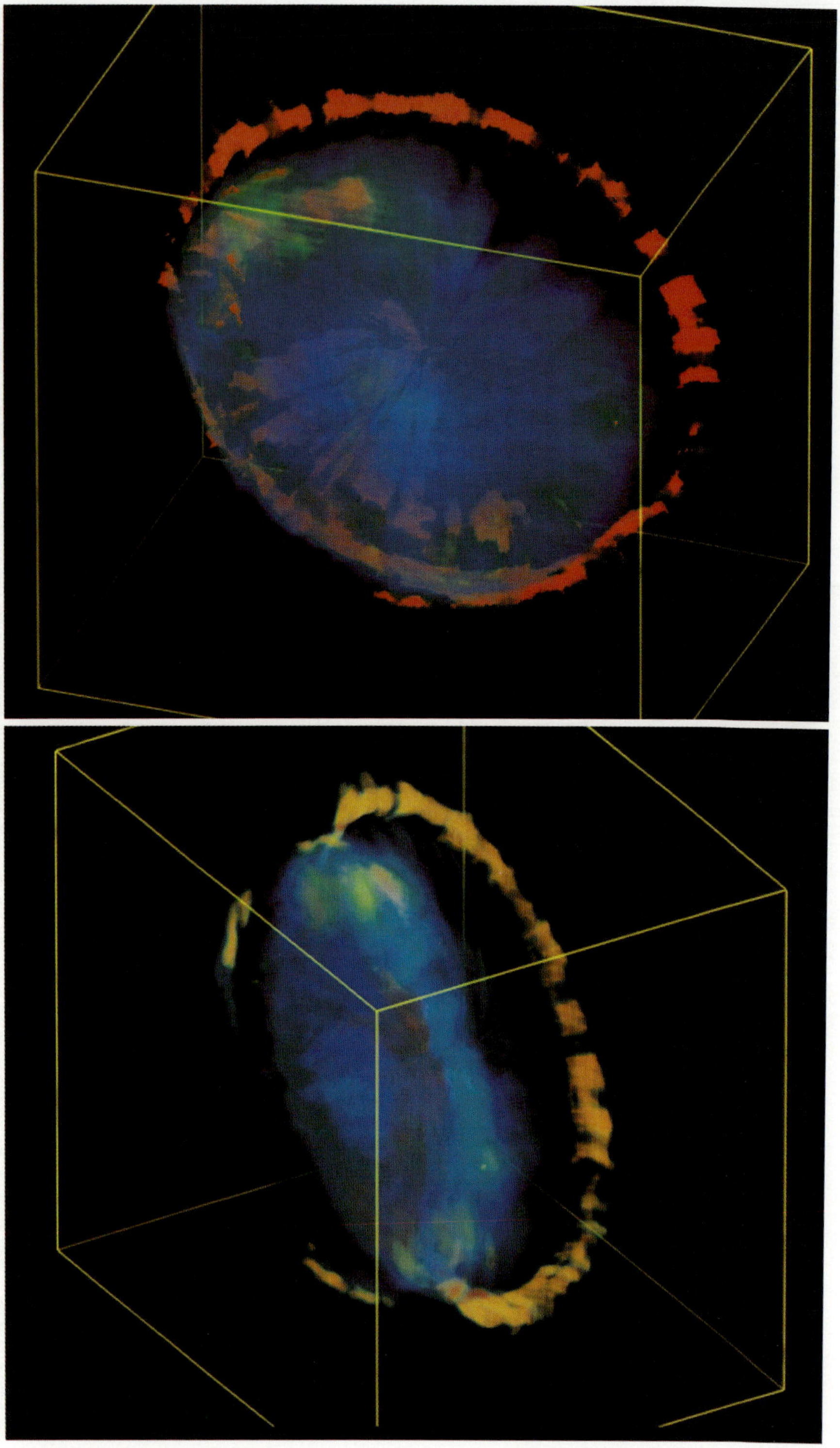

1c

1d

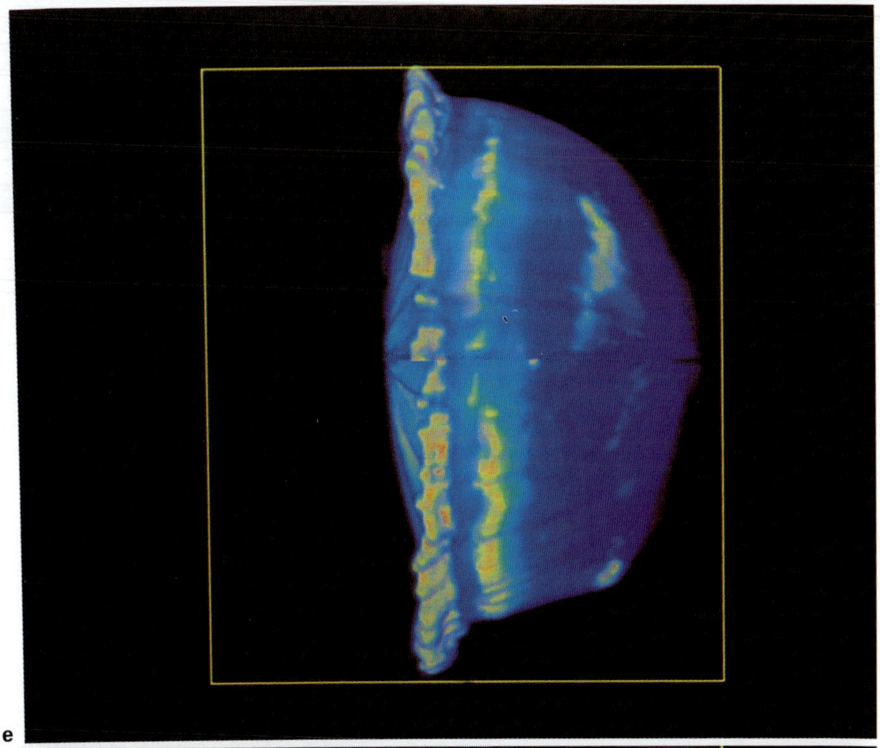

1e

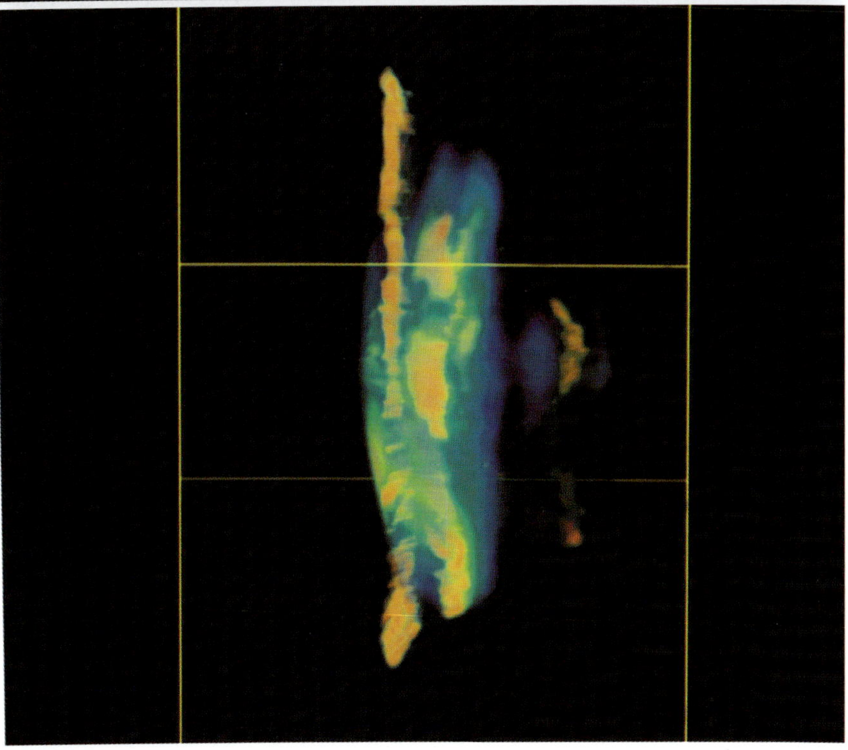

1f

bright voxels of the iris are orange. The volume rendering shown in figure 1e has been rotated on the optic axis to form that shown in figure 1f. Some of the voxels on the outer regions of the lens were made transparent in order that the regions of opacity in the deeper regions of the lens could be seen. This rendering shows regions of the cataract in the anterior and the posterior regions of the lens.

Discussion

The three-dimensional, pseudocolored rendering of the in vivo human ocular lens is an advance in the noninvasive techniques of three-dimensional ocular imaging. The visualization of the opacities of the human lens in three dimensions, with arbitrary cutting planes of any angle and direction, provides an improvement over the two-dimensional Scheimpflug images. Since the full volume of the ocular lens is available as a three-dimensional digital volume it can be viewed in any subregion and from any angle or viewpoint. The traditional Scheimpflug images are limited to information contained within the plane of the image. The use of pseudocoloring is helpful to visualize discrete regions of opacity in three-dimensions. Pseudocoloring is widely used in medical imaging, spacecraft imagery and satellite imaging, and airport X-ray machines to aid in the visualization of complex images [13].

The use of three-dimensional imaging and pseudocolor visualization of the in vivo human lens may be useful in the early detection of human cataracts. When applied to animal studies, these techniques may find application in ocular toxicity studies and the aging process of the lens.

Acknowledgements

This work was supported by NIH grant EY-06958 (B.R.M.).

References

1 Vogt A: Lehrbuch und Atlas der Spaltlampenmikroskopie des lebenden Auges. Berlin, Springer, 1930.
2 Berliner ML: Biomicroscopy of the Eye. New York, Hoebner, 1949, vol 2, p 927.
3 Oak SS, Laing RA, Neubauer L, Nogawa H, Majima Y: Clinical examination of the crystalline lens by retrocorneal specular microscopy. Ophthalmology 1983;90:346–351.
4 Bron AJ: Specular microscopy of human and animal lenses in vivo and vitro. Ophthalmology 1985;2:229–232.
5 Dragomirescu V, Hockwin O, Koch HR, Sasaki K: Development of a new equipment for rotating slit image photography according to Scheimpflug's principle. Interdiscipl Topics Gerontol 1978;13:1–13.
6 Hockwin O, Sasaki K, Lerman S: Evaluating cataract development with the Scheimpflug camera; in Masters BR (ed): Noninvasive Diagnostic Techniques in Ophthalmology, New York, Springer, 1990, pp 282–318.
7 Masters BR, Paddock SW: Three-dimensional reconstruction of the rabbit cornea by confocal scanning optical microscopy and volume rendering. Appl Optics 1990;29:3816–3822.
8 Masters BR, Farmer MF: Three-dimensional confocal microscopy and visualization of the in situ cornea. Comput Med Imaging Graph 1993;17:211–219.
9 Fitzke FW, Masters BR: Three-dimensional visualization of confocal sections of in vivo human fundus and optic nerve. Curr Eye Res 1993; 12:1015–1018.
10 Levoy M: Display of Surfaces from Volume Data. PhD dissertation. Chapel Hill, University of North Carolina at Chapel Hill, 1989.
11 Emori Y, Yasuda Y, Fukuda H, Sasaki S: Application of image processing technique for analyzing the optical system of the eye; in Fiorentini A, Guyton DL, Siegel IM (eds): Advances in Diagnostic Visual Optics. Berlin, Springer, 1987, pp 55–60.
12 Sakamoto Y, Sasaki K: Computed tomographic images and three-dimensional expression of crystalline lens findings from multiple slices of Scheimpflug slit images. Ophthalmic Res 1995;27(suppl 1):94–99.
13 Gonzales RC, Woods RE: Digital Image Processing. New York, Addison-Wesley Publishing, 1992, pp 237–242.

Ophthalmic Research

Ophthalmic Res 1996;28(suppl 2):127–130

Laser Scheimpflug Videography

H.-J. Huebscher[a]
D.E. Möller[a]
T. Seiler[b]

[a] Augenklinik im Klinikum Buch, Berlin, and
[b] Universitätsaugenklinik im UK CGC, Dresden, Germany

Key Words
Scheimpflug videographs
Laser illumination
Spatial resolution

Abstract
Conventional Scheimpflug photography uses slits with a constant width of 80 µm. This parameter limits the resolution as sharp contours are imaged with a basic uncertainty. In order to reduce this basic uncertainty we developed an illumination slit with a width of 20 µm and less, using a green helium-neon laser (543 nm). With this slit, much sharper imaging of ocular contours can be achieved. Since this illumination is coupled to on-line videographic detection of the Scheimpflug image, any adjustment of the target is done under visual control at the monitor. Using this device, the slope of a densitogram of contrasted contours (for example the corneal surfaces) is steeper, which guarantees a more accurate detection of corneal thickness and curvature.

Spatial resolution of conventional Scheimpflug records is limited by several factors, most of all by the optical slit width. In commercially available Scheimpflug systems the slit width amounts to 80 µm, thus leading to an uncertainty of the records of the same area (45° projection).

Further decrease of the slit width would result in a better spatial resolution; however, the image would be less bright and effects diffraction would increase. On the other hand, biometry of the anterior segment, including digital evaluation of curvatures, requires improved spatial resolution.

In this paper we describe the design of a laser system providing a substantial decrease of the slit width by means of optical imaging.

Material and Methods

Helium-neon laser continuously emitting at a wavelength of 543 nm was used. The constant power of the beam was 25 µW, which was increased during video recording to 500 µW for 0.1 s by means of a shutter mechanism.

KARGER

E-Mail karger@karger.ch
Fax + 41 61 306 12 34
http://www.karger.ch

© 1996 S. Karger AG, Basel
0030–3747/96/0288–0127$10.00/0

H.-J. Huebscher
Augenklinik im Klinikum Buch
Karower Strasse 11
D–13125 Berlin (Germany)

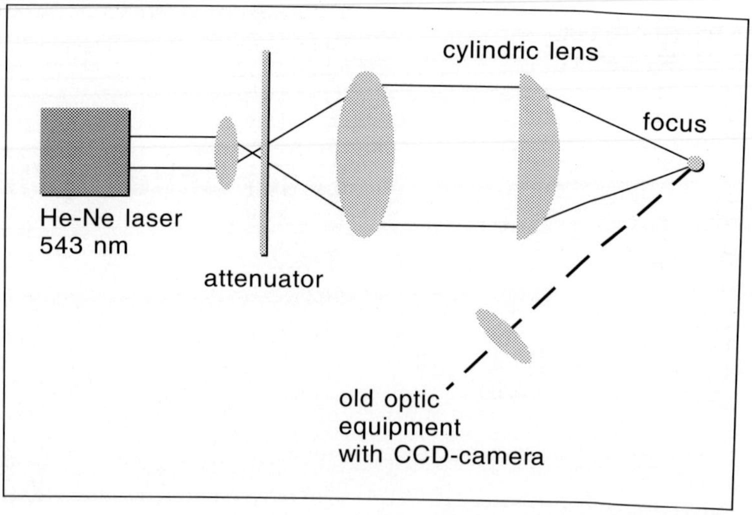

Fig. 1. Optics of the laser slit for Scheimpflug videography.

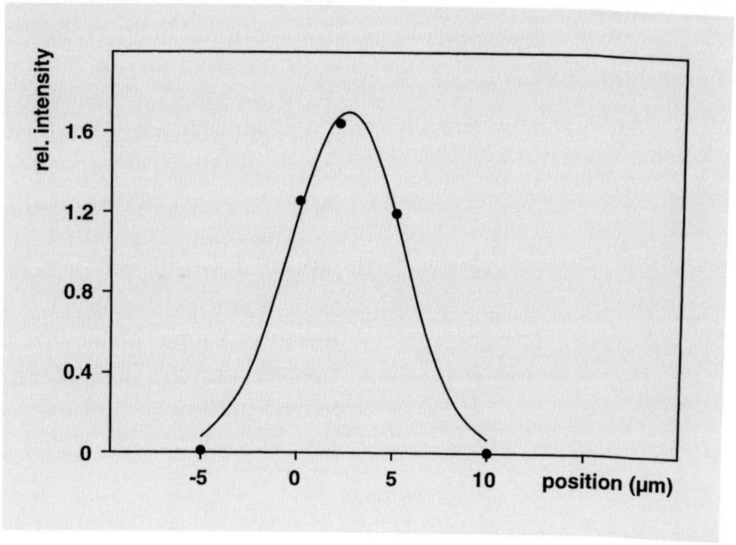

Fig. 2. Measurement of the laser beam width in the focus plane.

The circular laser beam was transformed to a slit by employing a cylindric lens with a focal length of 100 mm (fig. 1). In the focal plane, the slit line had a gaussian profile approximately 10 µm wide as determined by measurements using a pinhole diode (fig. 2). This width was obtained within a depth range of ± 0.3 mm around the focal plane.

For safety reasons, a constant illumination of the retina with a threshold power of 20 µW (line illumination) is legally considered not to be harmful (DIN VDE 0837, Tab VI). Assuming a pupil size of 7 mm, the maximal power at the retina is 10 µW in our case, well below the safety threshold. For pulsed laser light, the legal safety limit at 6 mJ is much higher than the 50 µJ created by our system. Thus, use of the laser in the mode described may be considered safe.

This illumination system was mounted in conjunction with the conventional CCD Scheimpflug camera recording path at an angle of 45°, fulfilling the Scheimpflug condition [1]. The continuous wave mode was used for aiming and adjusting, whereas the full beam pulsed mode was used for recording.

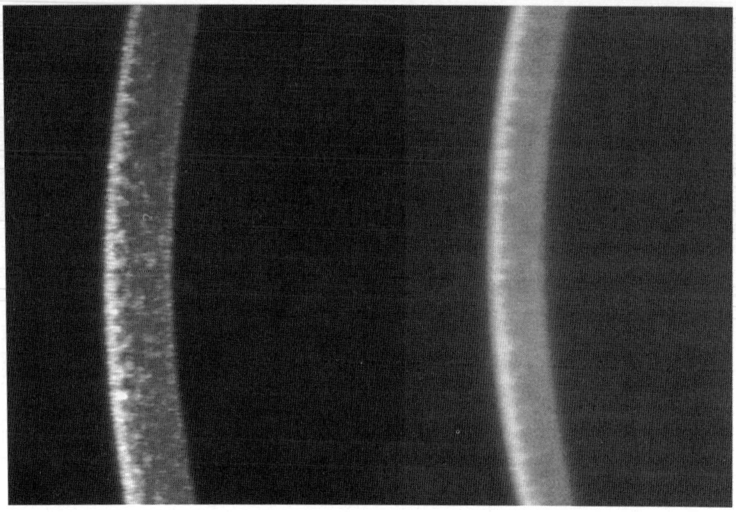

Fig. 3. Comparison of two Scheimpflug records from the same cornea. Right: with conventional illumination; left: with the new laser illumination system.

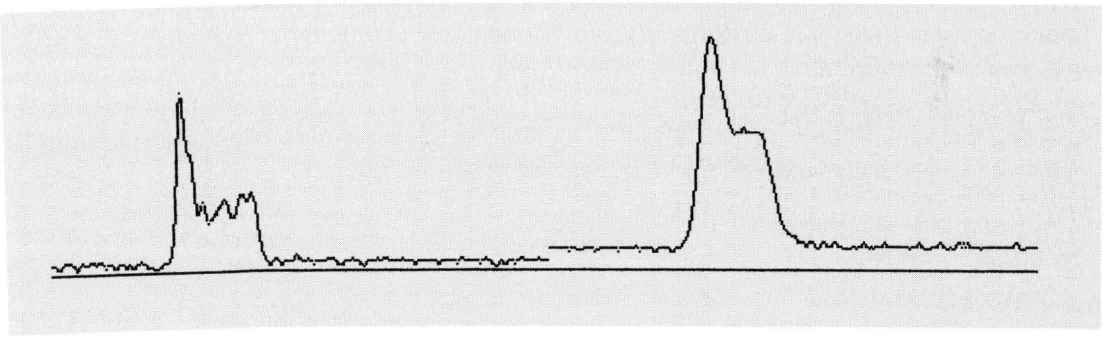

Fig. 4. Comparison of two densitograms. Right: from a cornea record with flash light illumination; left: a densitogram with laser illumination. The intrastromal structures represent uneven hydration.

Results

Figure 3 demonstrates a conventional flash light Scheimpflug videograph of a human cornea compared to a laser Scheimpflug videograph of the same eye. There is clearly less back-scattered light from the lens and iris, which results in a darker background and therefore in a better signal-to-noise ratio of the image.

Comparing densitograms using laser versus flash (fig. 4), it is obvious that the slopes of the front and rear surface of the cornea are much steeper and, consecutively, the location of the borders can be determined with better precision. Also, structures inside the cornea are sharper when detected in the laser densitogram as well as in the laser videograph, and less distinct in the flash record due to blurring. These scattering areas may originate from uneven hydration of the cornea.

Discussion

Until now, Scheimpflug photography was used in ophthalmology mainly for recording and measuring the clarity of the lens [2, 3]. For this application, photographic records using slits of 80 μm in width were sufficient and appropriate.

Recently, the Scheimpflug principle was also applied for biometry of the anterior segment, for example to measure the curvature of the corneal surfaces [4–6] as well as of the lens surface [7]. The precision of these measurements was rather limited by the spatial resolution of the recording systems, and to meet the demand for more precision, such as for the aspheric evaluation of the corneal curvature after refractive surgery, better illumination systems are required. An efficient way to overcome this problem is to use a laser beam optically transformed to a slit-like line.

This approach avoids diffractive problems, although slit widths of 20 μm and less are available (increasing the spatial resolution by a factor of 4). However, for this improvement a price must be paid: the depth of perception decreases to 1 mm and less, which is not an argument against corneal application, yet limits the application to the anterior segment as a whole. In addition, the substantially improved optical resolution can not be used in video-based recording systems unless the bandwidth of the video-electronic path of the system is increased. Currently bandwidths of 10 MHz are common, which is the reason for the partial loss of spatial resolution and information.

In summary, new applications of Scheimpflug photography require improved spatial resolution compared to commercially available systems. We demonstrated an alternative illumination system by using a laser beam that increased the precision and sharpness of the records.

References

1 Dragomirescu V, Sasaki K, Nakamura F, Hockwin O, Koch H-R, Kavasawa Y, Takizawa S: Rotating photo slit lamp based on Scheimpflug's principle. Digest Sci Pap 1st Symp Int Soc Ophthalmol Optics 1978;1:99–102.

2 Hockwin O, Dragomirescu V, Laser H: Measurements of lens transparency or its disturbances by densitometric image analysis of Scheimpflug-photographs. Graefe's Arch Clin Exp Ophthalmol 1983;219: 255–262.

3 Hockwin O, Dragomirescu V, Laser H, Wegener A, Eckerskorn U: Measuring lens transparency by Scheimpflug photography of the anterior eye segment: Principle, instrumentation and application to clinical and experimental ophthalmology. J Toxicol Cutan Ocul Toxicol 1987;6:251–271.

4 Richards DW, Russell SR, Anderson DR: A method for improved biometry of the anterior chamber with a Scheimpflug technique. Invest Ophthalmol Vis Sci 1988;29: 1826–1835.

5 Hachicha A, Simon S, Samson J, Hanna K: The use of gray-level information and fitting techniques for precise measurement of corneal curvature and thickness. Comput Vision Graph Image Process 1989;47: 165–188.

6 Seiler T, Huebscher H-J, Genth U: Corneal curvature change immediately after PRK as detected by Scheimpflug photography. Invest Ophthalmol Vis Sci 1993;34(suppl): 703.

7 Cook AC, Koretz JF: Acquisition of the curves of the human crystalline lens from slit lamp images: An application of the Hough transform. Appl Optics 1991;30:2088–2099.

Ophthalmic Research

Ophthalmic Res 1996;28(suppl 2):131–135

Molecular Masses of Gamma-Crystallins

M. Louise Riley[a]
John J. Harding[a]
Greg W. Kilby[b]
Roger J.W. Truscott[b]
Andrew Aquilina[b]
Margaret M. Sheil[b]

[a] Nuffield Laboratory of Ophthalmology, University of Oxford, UK;
[b] Australian Cataract Research Foundation, Department of Chemistry, University of Wollongong, Australia

Key Words
γ-Crystallins
Lens proteins
Electrospray mass spectrometry
Cataract

Abstract
Bovine γ-crystallins were isolated and analysed by electrospray mass spectrometry (ESMS). The mass of γII-crystallin was as predicted from the amino acid sequence and the mass of γIIIb-crystallin was close, but the mass of γIVa-crystallin was 59 Da greater than that expected. γIVa-Crystallin was digested with cyanogen bromide and the fragments were isolated before analysis by ESMS. The masses of the fragments did not correspond to the published sequence. The published sequence of γIVa-crystallin, which has been used to predict its three-dimensional structure, is incorrect.

Introduction

Structural changes in γ-crystallins occur during the development of cataract [1, 2]. γII-Crystallin has been used in numerous biophysical and chemical studies because its sequence is known and its three-dimensional structure has been determined to high resolution [3]. Its sequence was confirmed by electrospray mass spectrometry (ESMS) [4]. ESMS has been used to identify the mass and post-translational modifications of lens proteins [5].

γ-Crystallins have a molecular mass of approximately 21 kDa and a chain length of 173 or 174 residues [6]. The sequence of γIIIb-crystallin has been determined and correlated to the γD-crystallin gene [7]. Partial amino acid sequencing, X-ray diffraction data and extrapolation of sequences from the homologous rat γD- and γE-crystallins were used to predict the amino acid sequence of bovine γIVa-crystallin [8]. This sequence was used to build a three-dimensional model for γIVa-crystallin.

Bovine γ-crystallins were analysed by ESMS. The theoretical mass calculated from the sequence of γIVa-crystallin is 20,894 Da, which differs from the experimental mass obtained in this study (20,953 Da) by 59 Da. This discrepancy could be due to a single error in the sequence or to multiple errors. γIVa-Crystallin was digested with cyanogen bromide (CNBr) and the resulting fragments were analysed by ESMS.

KARGER

E-Mail karger@karger.ch
Fax + 41 61 306 12 34
http://www.karger.ch

© 1996 S. Karger AG, Basel
0030–3747/96/0288–0131$10.00/0

Dr. J.J. Harding
Nuffield Laboratory of Ophthalmology
University of Oxford
Walton Street
Oxford OX2 6AW (UK)

Materials and Methods

Nuclei from 12 bovine lenses were homogenized; then the γ-crystallins were separated from α- and β-crystallins by gel chromatography [9]. The individual γ-crystallins were then isolated [9]. γIVa-Crystallin was cleaved with CNBr [10] and the digest loaded onto a Sephadex G-50 gel filtration column (42 × 1 cm) at a flow rate of 3 ml/h with 100 m*M* acetic acid. Fractions of 1.25 ml were collected and the absorbance of each fraction was measured at 280 nm to locate the peptides. The eluted peptides were analysed by SDS-PAGE [11]. ESMS was as described [12].

Results

Total γ-crystallins were separated into γII-, γIII- and γIV-crystallin fractions using an SP-Sephadex C-50 column (elution profile not shown) [9] and were analysed by ESMS (table 1). The mass of γII-crystallin (20,969 Da), determined experimentally, is within 4 Da of the mass calculated from the reported sequence (20,965 Da) and that obtained previously by ESMS [4]. The theoretical mass of bovine γIIIa-crystallin was calculated as 20,743 Da and that of γIIIb-crystallin as 20,749 Da (table 1) from the sequences [7]. The ESMS of the γIII-crystallin fraction (not shown) shows a major peak at 20,748 Da,

Table 1. Calculated masses of bovine γ-crystallins from published sequences and masses determined experimentally by ESMS

	Calculated mass Da	Mass from ESMS Da
γII	20,965 [7]	20,969
γIIIa and	20,743	20,748
γIIIb	20,749 [7]	21,009
γIVa	20,894 [8]	20,953

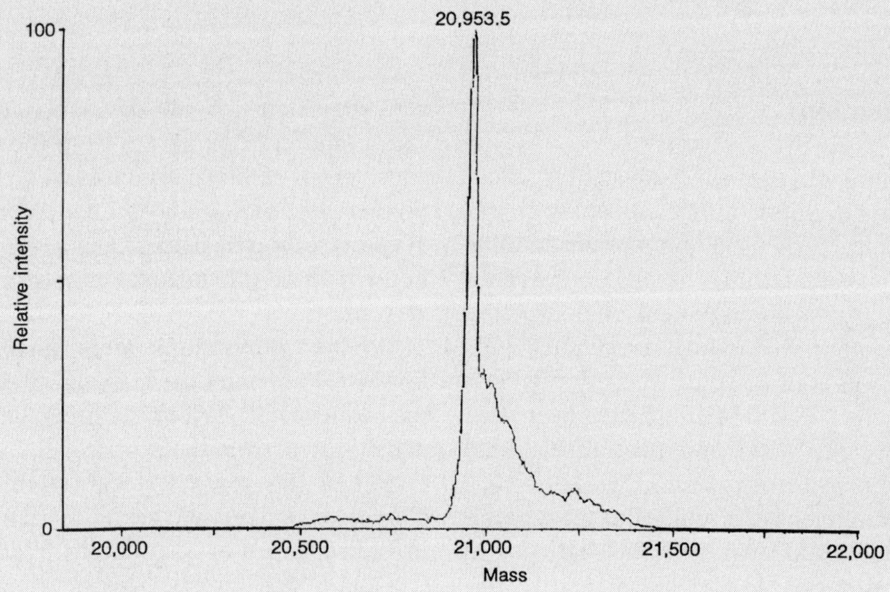

Fig. 1. ESMS of bovine γIV-crystallin.

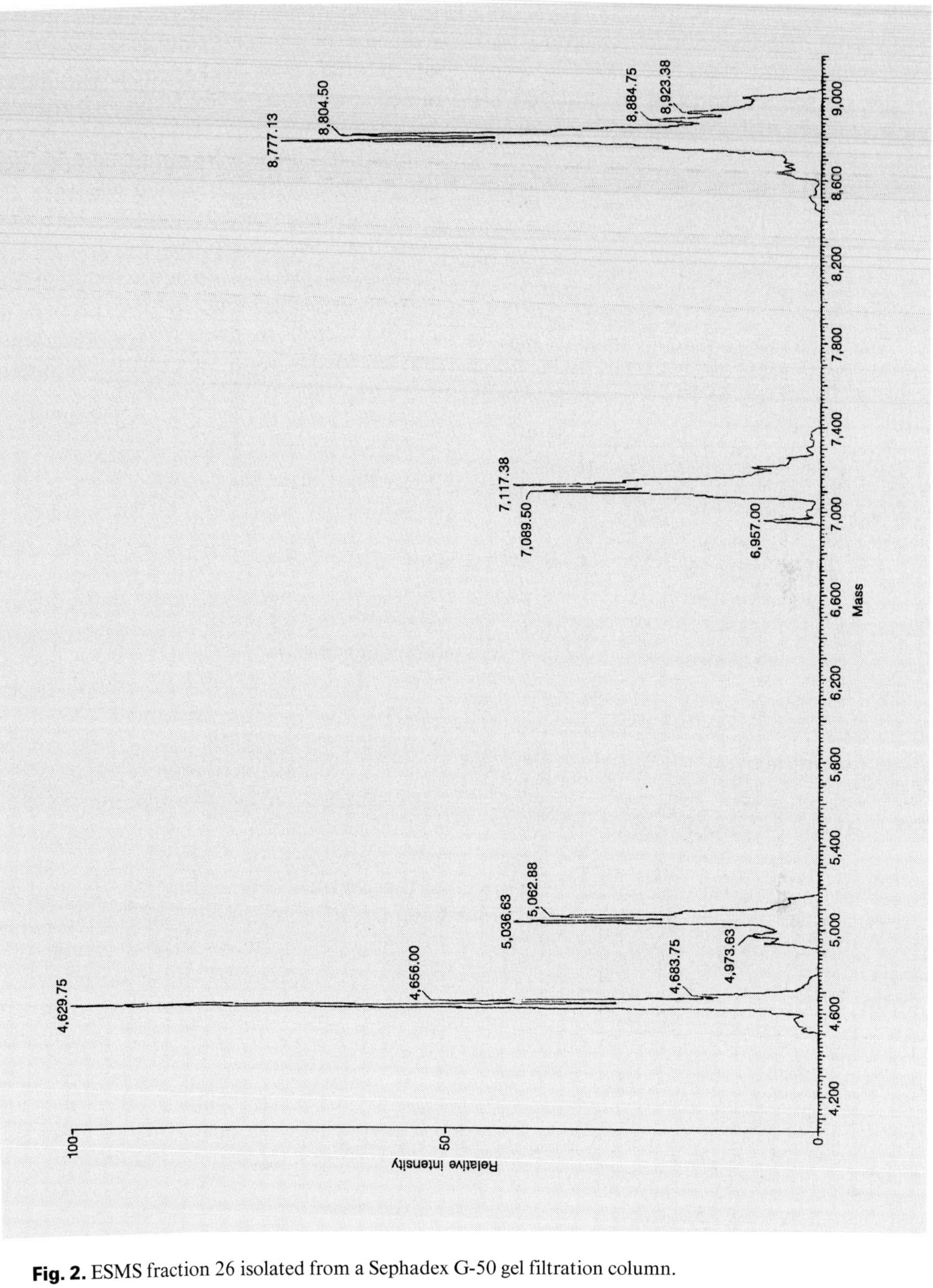

Fig. 2. ESMS fraction 26 isolated from a Sephadex G-50 gel filtration column.

which is close to the theoretical mass of both γIIIa- and γIIIb-crystallin. The second peak corresponded to a mass of 21,009 Da, which is 266 Da greater than OgIIIa- and 260 Da greater than γIIIb-crystallin. These results suggests that the published sequence of γIIIa-crystallin [7] does not correspond to the protein isolated from bovine lenses [12].

Table 2. Theoretical masses of CNBr peptides of bovine γIVa-crystallin calculated from the published sequence [8] and experimentally determined masses of CNBr cleavage products

Theoretical CNBr peptides (corrected for homoserine)	Mass of peptides (determined by ESMS)		
	fraction 25	fraction 26	fraction 27
From complete digestion			
1,159.2			
2,950.4			
3,288.5			
3,823.6			
4,548.5			
5,047.4			
From incomplete digestion			
4,121.6	4,172.4		4,417.5
	4,628.1	4,629.8	4,628.4
	4,654.6	4,656.0	4,655.8
			4,732.6
			4,792.1
	5,028.0		
	5,036.8	5,036.6	5,036.0
		5,062.9	5,064.9
5,719.7			
6,786.0			
	6,956.1		
	7,087.8	7,089.5	
7,124.1		7,117.4	
	7,185.0		
	7,230.6		
7,957.2			
8,349.0			
8,682.2			
	8,774.8	8,777.1	
	8,803.3	8,804.5	

The theoretical mass calculated from the sequence of γIVa-crystallin is 20,894 Da, which differs from the experimental mass obtained (20,953; fig. 1) by 59 Da. This discrepancy could not result from any likely post-translational modification but is more likely due to errors in the published sequence. Part of the sequence was determined by extrapolation from the homologous rat γD- and γE-crystallins [8] so it is not surprising that there may be errors present. γIVa-Crystallin was cleaved with CNBr, which splits the protein only on the carboxyl side of the methionine residues. Since γIVa-crystallin has 5 methionine residues in the published sequence [8], it would be expected to yield 6 peptides on reaction with CNBr. The cleavage products were separated partially before ESMS. Most of the cleaved products eluted in fractions 16–27 and were analysed by SDS-PAGE (not shown). Fractions 16–25 contained a mixture of partly cleaved peptides from 18 to 3 Da, indicating that incomplete digestion had occurred. Fractions 26 and 27 contained peptides from 6 to 2 kDa. Fractions 25, 26 and 27 were analysed by ESMS.

The ESMS of fraction 26 is shown in figure 2. The theoretical molecular masses of the 6 peptides expected if complete digestion of γIVa-crystallin had occurred, as well as some of the peptides expected as the result of incomplete digestion are shown in table 2. The experimental molecular masses obtained by ESMS do not agree with any of the theoretical values. These results indicate that there are several errors in the published sequence of γIVa-crystallin [8].

Discussion

The masses of γII- and γIIIb-crystallins obtained experimentally agree with the theoretical masses calculated from the published sequences to within a few daltons [7]. However the masses obtained for γIIIa- and γIVa-crystallin indicate that they have incorrect published sequences. γIVa-Crystallin was partially cleaved with CNBr into fragments, which werc analysed by ESMS. None of the masses matched those predicted from the published sequence, which has been used to model the three-dimensional structure of γIVa-crystallin [8]. Clearly the discrepancy in mass is not due to a single error. There must be multiple errors throughout the sequence.

Acknowledgements

We are grateful to RNIB and Research into Ageing for support.

References

1 Takemoto LJ, Hansen JS, Zigler JS, Horwitz J: Characterization of polypeptides from human nuclear cataracts by Western blot analysis. Exp Eye Res 1985;40:205–212.

2 Zigler JS, Russell P, Takemoto L, Schwab SJ, Hansen JS, Horwitz J, Kinoshita JH: Partial characterization of three distinct populations of human γ-crystallins. Invest Ophthalmol Vis Sci 1985;26:525–531.

3 Najmudin S, Nalini V, Driessen HPC, Slingsby C, Blundell TL, Moss DS, Lindley PF: Structure of bovine eye lens protein γB(γII)-crystallin at 1.47Å. Acta Crystallogr 1993;D49: 223–233.

4 Qin W, Smith JB, Smith DL: Reaction of aspirin with cysteinyl residues of lens γ-crystallins: A mechanism for the proposed anti-cataract effect of aspirin. Biochim Biophys Acta 1993;1181:103–110.

5 Kilby GW, Carver JA, Zhu JL, Sheil MM, Truscott RJW: Loss of the C-terminal serine residue from bovine pB2-crystallin. Exp Eye Res 1995; 60:465–469.

6 Harding JJ: Cataract: Biochemistry, Epidemiology and Pharmacology. London, Chapman & Hall, 1991.

7 Hay RE, Andley UP, Petrash JM: Expression of recombinant bovine γB-, γC- and γD-crystallin and correlation with native proteins. Exp Eye Res 1994;58:573–584.

8 White HE, Driessen HPC, Slingsby C, Moss DS, Lindley PF: Packing interactions of the eye-lens: Structural analysis, internal symmetry and lattice interactions of bovine γIVa-crystallin. J Mol Biol 1989; 207:217–235.

9 Martin S, Harding JJ: Site of carbamylation of bovine γII-crystallin by potassium [^{14}C] cyanate. Biochem J 1989;262:909–915.

10 Panjwani NA, Harding JJ: Isolation and hydroxylysine glycoside content of some cyanogen bromide-cleaved fragments of collagen from bovine corneal stroma. Biochem J 1978; 171:687–695.

11 Swank RT, Munkres KD: Molecular weight analysis of oligopeptides by electrophoresis in polyacrylamide gel with sodium dodecyl sulfate. Anal Biochem 1971;39:462–477.

12 Kilby GW, Truscott RJW, Aquilina JA, Sheil MM, Riley ML, Harding JJ: Electrospray ionisation mass spectrometry of lens crystallins: Verification and detection of errors in protein sequences of bovine γ-crystallins. Eur Mass Spectrom 1995;1: 203–208.

Ophthalmic Research

Ophthalmic Res 1996;28(suppl 2):136–140

M. Nagata[a,c]
M. Kojima[a]
H. Murano[a]
K. Sasaki[a]
Y. Obara[b]
K. Matsuura[c]
H. Takashina[c]

Distributional Change of Alpha-Tocopherol in the Rat Lens with Age

[a] Department of Ophthalmology, Kanazawa Medical University, Ishikawa, and
[b] Department of Ophthalmology, Dokkyo Koshigaya Hospital, Dokkyo University School of Medicine, Saitama, and
[c] Developmental Laboratories, Santen Pharmaceutical Co., Ltd., Osaka, Japan

Key Words
d-α-Tocopherol
Vitamin E
Lens
Brown-Norway rat
Gas chromatography mass spectrometry (GC/MS)

Abstract

Concentration of α-tocopherol (α-Toc.) in the rat lens (1, 4 and 12 months old) was determined in single lenticular layers using gas chromatography and mass spectrometry. The highest concentration of α-Toc. in lens was found in the nucleus, followed by the deeper anterior and deeper posterior cortices, the shallow anterior and shallow posterior cortices, and the equatorial region. The topographic α-Toc. distribution in the lens did not differ between lenses of 1-, 4- and 12-month-old rats. A significant decrease of α-Toc. concentration was seen in lenses of 4- and 12-month-old rats compared to those 1 month old. Concentration and distribution in 4- and 12-month-old rat lenses were almost the same. The concentration of α-Toc. in the lens changes in relation to age.

Introduction

Oxidation of lenticular proteins has been recognized as a major causative factor in so-called age-related cataract [1], and cataract risk might be modified by intake of antioxidant nutrients such as vitamin C [2–10], α-tocopherol (α-Toc.) [11–15] and carotenoid [8]. α-Toc. has been thought to play an important role in protecting polyunsaturated fatty acid from oxidative damage [16]. Concentration of α-Toc. in the lenses has been measured by high-performance liquid chromatography [16, 17]. However, the total amount of α-Toc. is quite low in the lens [16]. Although the topographic distribution of α-Toc. in single len-

KARGER

E-Mail karger@karger.ch
Fax + 41 61 306 12 34
http://www.karger.ch

© 1996 S. Karger AG, Basel
0030–3747/96/0288–0136$10.00/0

Masami Kojima, PhD
Department of Ophthalmology
Kanazawa Medical University
1-1 Daigaku, Uchinada
Ishikawa 920-02 (Japan)

ticular layers is of interest in correlation to the formation of cataract types, the method of α-Toc. determination mentioned above is not sensitive enough to measure the concentration of α-Toc. in single layers of the lens.

This study was designed to examine the topographic distribution of α-Toc. in the lens using gas chromatography and mass spectrometry (GC/MS).

Material and Methods

Lens Preparation

One-, 4-, and 12- month-old Brown-Norway rats (n = 5 rats in each group) were used in this study. Rat lenses were dissected from freshly enucleated eyes and divided into the equatorial ring (20% of lenticular diameter) and the inner cylinder (80% of lenticular diameter) with 2.5 mm (for 1-month-old rats) and 3.0 mm (for 4- and 12-month-old rats) trepan. Lenticular layers were sliced at thicknesses of 0.05 mm (for 1-month-old rats) and 0.75 mm (for 4- and 12-month-old rats) from the anterior to the posterior side of the inner cylinder with BONN microsectioning equipment at –6 °C [18, 19], obtaining 6 single lenticular regions (fig. 1). In order to provide enough material for test preparation, the corresponding lenticular layers of 2 lenses in a rat were pooled to give 1 analytical sample. These layers were weighed, and stored at –80 °C before α-Toc. measurement.

GC/MS Analysis of α-Toc

Lenticular samples were homogenized and α-Toc. was extracted with n-hexane. The organic phase was further extracted with Bond Elut SI, and α-Toc. was esterized with pentafluoropropionic anhydride. Electron ionization and selected ion monitoring were used in the GC/MS system (fig. 2).

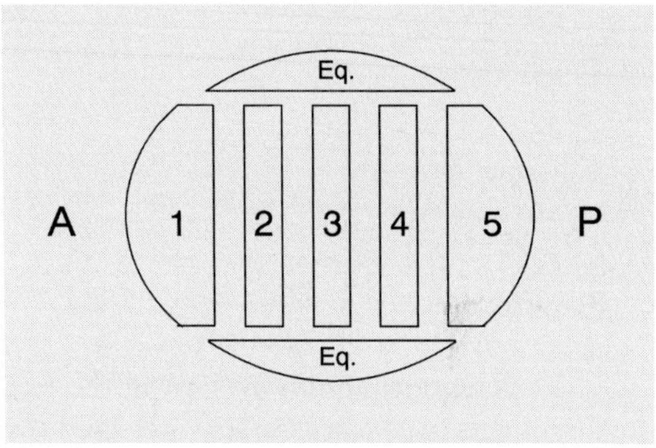

Fig. 1. Diagram of lens sectioning. A = Anterior part; P = posterior part; Eq.= equator.

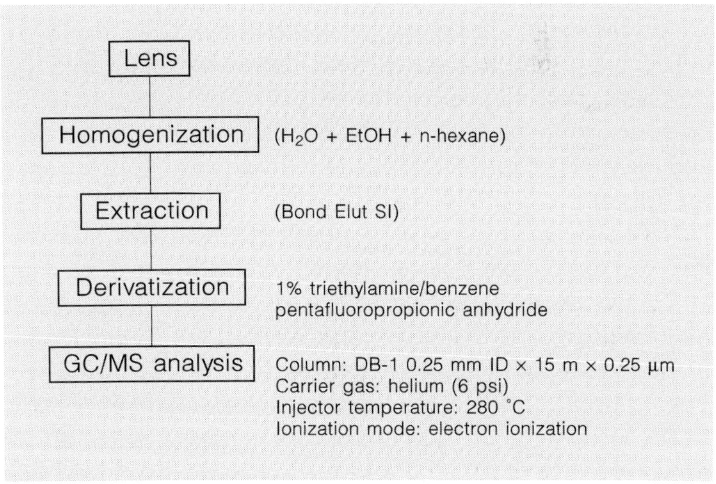

Fig. 2. Procedure for determination of α-Toc. in lenticular sections.

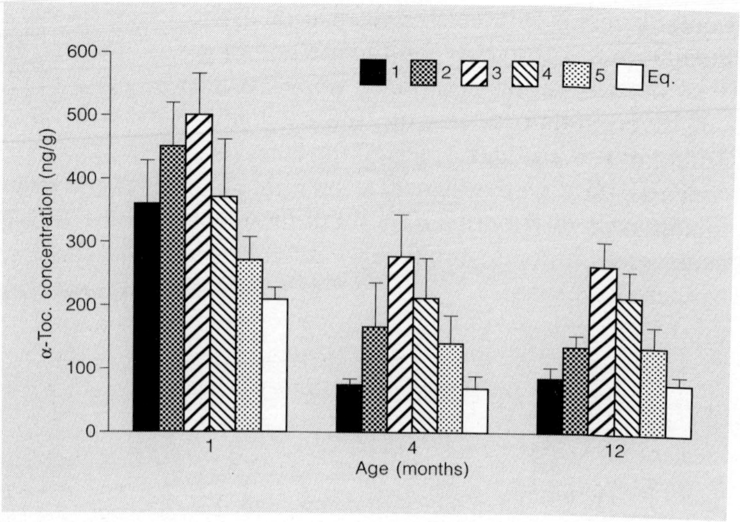

Fig. 3. Age-related topographic distributional changes of α-Toc. in the single lenticular layers. 1 = Shallow anterior cortex; 2 = deeper anterior cortex; 3 = nucleus; 4 = deeper posterior cortex; 5 = shallow posterior cortex; Eq. = equator. Data represents mean ± SD (n = 5).

Results

The concentration of α-Toc. from the lenticular layers was successfully detected by GC/MS. The highest concentration of α-Toc. in 1-month-old rat lens was in the nuclear region followed by the deeper anterior cortex, the deeper posterior cortex, the shallow anterior cortex, the shallow posterior cortex, and the equatorial region. The α-Toc. distribution patterns from 4- and 12-month-old lens were almost the same. The highest concentration of α-Toc. was found in the nucleus followed by the deeper posterior cortex, the deeper anterior cortex and the shallow posterior cortex, and the shallow anterior cortex and the equator (fig. 3).

α-Toc. concentration of 4-month-old rat lens was lower than that of 1-month-old rats and about the same as that of 12-month-old rat lenses in every section. To compare with 1- and 4-month-old rat lenses in each section, α-Toc. concentration in the shallow anterior cortex (section 1) of 4-month-old rat lenses was one fourth of 1-month-old rat lenses. α-Toc. concentration in the other sections of 4-month-old rat lenses was between one third and one half that of 1-month-old rats (fig. 3).

Discussion

Many studies deal with the relationship between serum α-Toc. level and cataract [8, 11, 20–22]. Some reported a positive relation between serum α-Toc. level and cataract prevalence [8, 11, 20], and others found no correlation [21, 22]. Studies of a correlation between lenticular α-Toc. concentration and cataract formation are few [16, 23], and their conclusions also differ. Dillon et al. [23] could not find a significant change of lenticular α-Toc. concentration with formation of cataract. In contrast, Bessems et al. [16] found a significant difference of α-Toc. proportion between lenses with nuclear cataract and normal lenses. Their possible explanation for the difference between their results and those of Dillon et al. [23] was that the latter data were from mixed-type cataract (both cortical and nuclear opacities existed in 1 lens), and that they did not distinguish between lenticular regions. If one converts the region-specific data of Bessems et al. into the whole-lens data, they agree with the findings of Dillon et al., which indicates that a whole-lens study is inadequate to evaluate such small lenticular changes. For this reason we evaluated lenticular α-Toc. distribution in single lenticular layers with GC/MS.

In this study, we found that the concentration of α-Toc. in the rat lens fell dramatically at the age of 4 months compared to at 1 month, and that the amount and distribution pattern of α-Toc. were the same as at 12 months of age. The reduction of the α-Toc. concentration at 1 and 4 months of age seems to correlate with the normal lenticular growth. The wet weight of rat lenses increases linearly at approximately 3–4 months of age; then the rate of increase is gradually reduced and after 1.5 years of age it becomes almost stable [24]. In a comparison of α-Toc. concentrations in 1- and 4-month-old single lenticular layers, we observed the interesting phenomenon that the concentration in the shallow anterior cortex of 4-month-old rat lenses was one fifth that of 1-month-old rat lenses, while its concentration in the nuclear region was more than one half (fig. 3). The reason for the lenticular-region-dependent α-Toc. difference is unclear.

α-Toc. will be used to prevent membrane oxidation mainly in the anterior part of lens, especially the lenticular epithelium and remnant α-Toc. of the anterior part of the lens stored in the lenticular nuclear area.

Liebler et al. [25] reported that α-Toc. suppressed lipid oxyradical propagation, which was measured as malondialdehyde production. Moreover, α-Toc. prevents oxidation of phospholipid bilayers, and prevention of membrane phospolipid peroxidation by α-Toc. causes stabilization of lenticular membranes.

Acknowledgement

The excellent technical assistance of Ms. Yukari Midori is greatly appreciated.

References

1 Vision Research, a National Plan: The Report of the Cataract Panel (NIH publication 83-2473). Washington, US Department Health Human Services, 1983, vol 2, part 3.

2 Ogino S, Yasukura K: Biochemical studies on cataract. VI. Production of cataratcs in guinea pigs with dinitrophenol. Am J Ophthalmol. 1957; 43:936–946.

3 Kosegarten DC, Maher TJ: Use of guinea pig as model to study galactose-induced cataract formation. J Pharm Sci 1987;67:1478–1479.

4 Varma SD, Srivastava VK, Richards RD: Photooxidation in lens and cataract formation – Preventive role of superoxide dismutase, catalase and vitamin C. Ophthalmic Res 1982;14:167–175.

5 Nishigori H, Hayashi R, Lee JW, Murayama K, Iwatsuru M: Preventive effect of ascorbic acid against glucocorticoid-induced cataract formation of developing chick embryos. Exp Eye Res 1985;40: 445–451.

6 Vinson JA, Possanza CJ, Drack AV: The effect of ascorbic acid on galactose-induced cataracts. Nutr Rep Int 1986;33:665–668.

7 Blondin J, Baragi V, Schwartz E, Sadowski J, Taylor A: Delay of UV-induced eye lens protein damage in guinea pig by dietary ascorbate. J Free Radic Biol Med 1986;2:275–281.

8 Jacques PF, Hartz SC, Chylack LT, McGandy RB, Sadwski JA: Nutritional status in persons with and without senile cataract – Blood vitamin and mineral levels. Am J Clin Nutr 1988;48:152–158.

9 Nagata M, Tanioka H, Mibu H, Hikida M, Akiba M, Yamamoto I: Effect of ascorbic acid 2-O-α-glucoside on hydrocortisone-induced cataract formation in developing chick embryos. I. Comparison of the preventive effect of ascorbic acid derivates. J Ocul Pharmacol 1993;9:59–68.
10 Nagata M, Hikida M, Mibu H, Muto N, Yamamoto I: Effect of ascorbic acid 2-O-α-glucoside on hydrocortisone-induced cataract formation in developing chick embryos. II. Influence on glutathione and lipid peroxide contents in the lens. J Ocul Pharmacol 1994;10:537–542.
11 Robertson JM, Donner AP, Trevithick JR: Vitamin E intake and risk of cataracts in humans. Ann NY Acad Sci 1989;570:372–382.
12 Creighton MO, Trevithick JR: Cortical cataract formation prevented by vitamin E and glutathione. Exp Eye Res 1979;29:689–693.
13 Varma SD, Beachy NA, Richards RD: Photoperoxidation of lens lipids – Prevention by vitamin E. Photochem Photobiol 1982;36:623–636.
14 Creighton MO, Ross WM, Stewart-DeHaan PJ, Sanwal M, Trevithick JR: Modeling cortical cataractogenesis. VII. Effects of vitamin E treatment on galactose-induced cataracts. Exp Eye Res 1985;40:213–222.
15 Tappel AL: Vitamin E and selenium protection from in vivo lipid peroxidation. Ann NY Acad Sci 1980; 3555:18–31.
16 Bessems GJH, Man BM, Hoenders HJ, Wollensak J: Alpha-tocopherol in the normal and nuclear-cataractous human lens. Lens Res 1984–1985;2:233–242.
17 Hirai T, Majima Y, Ohta Y, Ishiguro I: Antioxidative role of vitamin E in rabbit lens. J Eye 1985;2:1174–1177.
18 Müller A, Möller B, Dragomirescu V, Hockwin O: Profiles of enzyme activities in bovine lenses; in Hockwin O (ed): Drug-Induced Ocular Side Effects and Ocular Toxicology. Concepts Toxicol. Basel, Karger 1987, vol 4,pp 343–349.
19 Kojima M: Enzymatic distribution patterns of rat lenses and the changes that occur during naphthalene caract development. Ophthalmic Res 1992;24:73–82.
20 Knect P, Heliovaara M, Rissanen A, Aromaa A, Aaran RK: Serum antioxidant vitamins and risk of cataract. BMJ 1992;305:1392–1394.
21 Costagliola C, Iuliano G, Menzione M, Nesti A, Simonelli F, Rinalidi E: Systemic human diseases as oxidative risk factors in cataractogenesis. Ophthalmic Res 1988;20:308–316.
22 Vatassery GT, Johnson GJ, Krezowski AM: Changes in vitamin E concentrations in human plasma and platelets with age. J Am Coll Nutr 1983;4:369–375.
23 Dillon J, Mehlman B, Ponticorvo L, Spector A: The stage of neutral lipids in normal and cataractous human lenses. Exp Eye Res 1983;37:91–98.
24 Von Heyningen R: Biochemistry of the lens; in Perkins ES, Hill DW (eds): Scientific Foundations of Ophthalmology, London, Heinemann, 1976.
25 Liebler DC, Kling DS, Reed DJ: Antioxidant protection of phospholipid bilayer by α-tocopherol. J Biol Chem 1986;261:12114–12119.

Author Index

Numbers refer only to this Supplement Issue

Subject Index

Numbers refer only to this Supplement Issue

Epidemiology of Blindness and Eye Disease

Editors:
H.G. Krumpaszky, V. Klauß

Provides a comprehensive survey of the causes of blindness over the past century and important insights into the results of present epidemiological research on eye diseases

Contents

Introduction
- Historical Aspects
- Objectives of the Study

Materials and Methods
- Research Strategy
- Evaluation
- Evolutionary Trends
- Classification of the Causes of Blindness
- Determining the Cause of Blindness
- Definitions of Blindness
- Material for Studies on the Number of Blind and the Causes of Blindness

Results
- Blindness Rate in Germany
- Number of Visually Handicapped
- Degree of Disability
- Demographics of the Onset Blindness
- Sex Distribution
- Age Distribution
- Age at the Onset of Blindness
- Duration of Blindness
- Macular Degeneration as a Cause of Blindness
- Diabetes Mellitus as a Cause of Blindness
- Cataract as a Cause of Blindness
- Glaucoma as a Cause of Blindness
- High-Grade Myopia as a Cause of Blindness
- Retinal Detachment as a Cause of Blindness
- 'Tapetoretinal' Degeneration (Retinitis Pigmentosa) as a Cause of Blindness
- Optic Atrophy (Degeneration of the Optic Nerve) as a Cause of Blindness
- Infections as Causes of Blindness
- Disorders of the Uvea as a Cause of Blindness
- Injuries as a Cause of Blindness

Blindness in Childhood
- Prevalence and Incidence of Childhood Blindness
- Bupthalmia as a Cause of Blindness
- Congenital Cataract as a Cause of Blindness
- Malformations as Causes of Blindness
- Retinopathy of Prematury as a Cause of Blindness
- Amblyopia in Childhood

Ophthalmologica
Editor: Ohrloff, Ch. (Frankfurt)
ISSN 0030–3755
Special issue: Vol. 210, No. 1 (1996)
Included in subscription

Epidemiology of Blindness and Eye Disease
Editors: Krumpaszky, H.G. (Tübingen); Klauß, (München)
84 p., 191 tab., soft cover, 1996
CHF 80.– / DEM 96.– / USD 69.75
Prices subject to change
DEM price for Germany, USD price for USA only
ISBN 3–8055–6315–9

Fields of Interest: Ophthalmology; Epidemiology; Social and Preventive Medicine

KI 96461

KARGER

Indispensable for Ophthalmologists

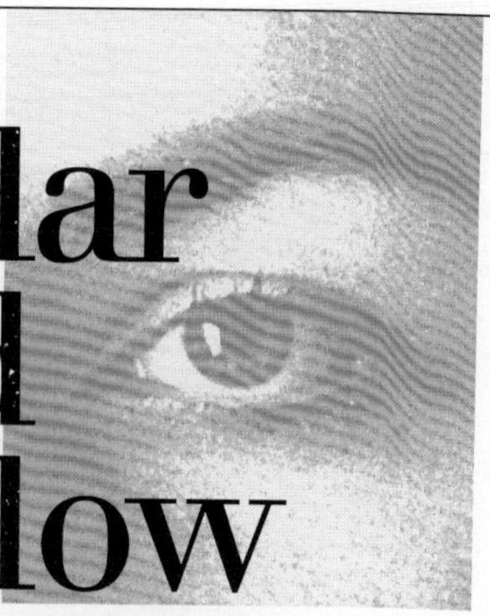

Ocular Blood Flow

New Insights into the Pathogenesis of Ocular Diseases

Editors: H. J. Kaiser, J. Flammer, Ph. Hendrickson

This book is a synopsis of up-to-date knowledge on the quantification of ocular blood perfusion and originates from expert lectures held at the 1995 Glaucoma Meeting in Switzerland. In the first section, a profound overview of the anatomy, physiology and pathophysiology of ocular perfusion enables the reader to gain distinct new insights into the pathogenesis of ocular diseases. The second part of the publication describes the different measuring methods that are currently applied in clinical practice and in research. It has been written by a team of leading researchers with the aim of bringing their findings to the attention of those working directly with patients, in particular the ophthalmologist in the clinic or private practice.

Contents

Büchi, E.R.: The Blood Supply to the Optic Nerve Head
Nicholls, J.G.: Regrowth of Nerve Fibers and Recovery of Function after Spinal Injury
Flammer, J.: To What Extent Are Vascular Factors Involved in the Pathogenesis of Glaucoma?
Pournaras, C.J.: Autoregulation of Ocular Blood Flow
Haefliger, I.O.; Meyer, P.; Flammer, J.; Lüscher, T.F.: Endothelium-Dependent Vasoactive Factors
Meyer, P.; Haefliger, I.O.; Flammer, J.; Lüscher, T.F.: Endothelium-Dependent Regulation in Ocular Vessels
Haefliger, I.O.; Anderson, D.R.: Pericytes and Capillary Blood Flow Modulation
Cioffi, G.A.; Orgül, S.: Intraluminal Corrosion Casting and Colored-Microsphere Techniques as Means to Assess Optic Nerve Hemodynamics
Orgül, S.; Cioffi, G.A.: The Vasomotor Effect of Arterial Oxygen on the Optic Nerve Microvasculature
Bebie, H.: Introduction to the Doppler Effect
Lieb, W.E.: Color Doppler Imaging of the Orbit
Kaiser, H.J.: Color Doppler Imaging in Glaucoma Patients
Petrig, B.L.; Riva, C.E.: Optic Nerve Head Laser Doppler Flowmetry: Principles and Computer Analysis
Riva, C.E.; Mendel, M.; Petrig, B.L.: Flicker-Induced Optic Nerve Blood Flow Change
Pillunat, L.E.; Anderson, D.R.; Knighton, R.W.; Joos, K.M.; Feuer, W.J.: Effect of Increased Intraocular Pressure on Optic Nerve Head Blood Flow
Stock, K.W.: Basic Principles of Magnetic Resonance Imaging
Stock, K.W.: Magnetic Resonance Angiography: Technique and Clinical Applications in the Carotid Region
Mattle, H.P.: Detection of Cerebral Ischemia with Magnetic Resonance
Rudin, M.; Beckmann, N.; Bruttel, K.; Markstein, R., Prünte, C.: Measurement of Tissue Perfusion Using Magnetic Resonance Imaging: Assessment of Drug Effects on Optic Nerve Perfusion in Rats
Bischoff, P.M.: Basic Principles of Choroidal Angiography and Its Possible Applications
Prünte, C.: Indocyanine Green Angiography in Patients with Normal-Tension Glaucoma
Ulrich, A.: Choroidal Angiography with Perfusion Pressure Videoangiography
Nasemann, J.E.; Carl, T.; Spiegel, D.: Measurement of Systemic and Ocular Blood Flow Velocities in Normal-Tension Glaucoma
Drance, S.M.: In Light of New Findings, How Do We Manage Open-Angle Glaucoma Patients in 1995?

Ocular Blood Flow
New Insights into the Pathogenesis of Ocular Diseases
Glaucoma Meeting, Basel, March 1995
Editors: Kaiser, H.J.; Flammer, J.; Hendrickson, P. (Basel)
VIII + 226 p., 106 fig., 19 in color, 12 tab., hard cover, 1996
CHF 167.– / DEM 200.– / USD 145.25
Prices subject to change
DEM price for Germany, USD price for USA only
ISBN 3–8055–6238–1

Field of Interest: Ophthalmology

KI 96440

KARGER